SECRET OF HEALTH

By

Pt. Ravinder Lakhotia

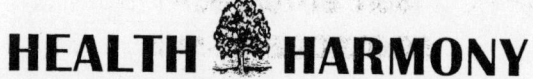

SECRET OF HEALTH

Reprint Edition: 2006

No part of this book may be reproduced, stored in a retrieval system or transmitted, in any form or by any means, mechanical, photocopying, recording or otherwise, without any prior written permission of the Publishers.

© Copyright with the Publishers.

Price: Rs. 50.00

Published by Kuldeep Jain for

HEALTH HARMONY

an imprint of **B. Jain Publishers (P) Ltd.**
1921, Street No. 10, Chuna Mandi,
Paharganj, New Delhi 110 055 (INDIA)
Phones: 91-011-2358 0800, 2358 1100, 2358 1300, 2358 3100
Fax: 91-011-2358 0471; *Email:* bjain@vsnl.com
Website: **www.bjainbooks.com**

Printed in India by
J.J. Offset Printers
522, FIE, Patpar Ganj, Delhi - 110 092
Phones: 91-011-2216 9633, 2215 6128

ISBN: 81-7021-967-1
BOOKCODE: BL-5435

Contents

Preface .... ( )
Foreward .... (v)
Introduction .... (vii)
Mind and Disease 1
How to be Happy 4
Karma and Yog 7
Mantra 12
Mental Crime 14
Behaviour 16
Protection of Babies & Animals 23
Knowledge of Personalities 29
Invaluable Knowledge 33
Relations 44
Tension 46
Dhyan and Yoga 50
Indian Ayurvedic Massage 61
Mudra Therapy 67
Reiki 75
Crystal Healing 78
Miracles of Science (Dowsing) 83
Insomnia (Sleeplessness) 85
Food 90
Flower Therapy 105
Summary 108

PREFACE

First of all I bow my head before the deity of Lord Ganesha, Maa Laxmi and Maa Bhagwati. Thereafter I express gratitude to my parents who inspired me to write this book. I dedicate this books to my Hon'ble Guruji Swami Omkarananda ji, Swami Vishveshwarananda Ji, Swami Soma Shekhari ji, Swami Gori Shankarananda ji, Swami Sachidananda ji, Swami Vishwaroopa ji, Swami Narsinghmullu ji and Swami Usha Ji (Omkarananda Ashram Himalyas) Acharya Mahapragya ji, Yuwacharya Mahasharman ji, Swami Purshotam Dass Ji, Mrs. Paula Horen (Reiki Master, USA), Dr. Taru Bhagat, I extend my thanks to Hon'ble Sh. Yogesh Sachdeva Ji, Smt. Kusum Tantia, Sh. Bansilal Ji Rathi, Mrs. & Mr. U.G.S. Rao, Kuldeep Jain, R.P. Jain, Sanjay Jain, Hema & Sangita Lakhotio who have guided from time to time and extended their valuable contribution to this manuscript.

FOREWORD

I have been assigned to translate this book on supernatural therapy written by Pt. Ravinder Lakhotia in english. I found the book very useful in daily life.

Human beings have made their life so busy that when they fall sick they take resort in allopathy. Despite spending a huge amount, they gain nothing. After going from pillar to post one meets a man like Pt. Ravinder Lakhotia who then advises natural/supernatural therapy which is mentioned in this book and most of the people are relieved by adopting the suggested therapy. I feel, disorders in the body are our own faults as we do not care about environmental behaviors and act against the rules of nature. If one goes by the rules of nature, maintains brotherhood and never thinks ill of others, he will remain hale and hearty. On account of any mistake or lapse, if any disease occurs, he should revert back to his natural path as suggested in this book. This is the gist which the author wants to convey. I hope this book is helpful to those who trust God and nature.

I have made a very humble attempt to translate the book verbatim. I will be happy if any error is pointed out by any reader.

I again thank the author who has given me a chance to do this noble work.

R.P. Jain
Advocate
Bhiwani
1.7.99

INTRODUCTION

In today's modern and competitive life, human beings are occupied to such an extent that it seems difficult for them to even spare 15 minutes a day for study. If it so happens, then besides enriching our knowledge it will prove to be our best guide.

This books does not contain any preaching. Rather it contains the practical knowledge of assessing an individual, strengthening the relations and to remove tension from daily life for which everyone gives and will like to give recognition. This book is useful for all, children, young and old.

Pandit Ravinder Lakhotia
(Super–natural Healer, Numerologist, Dowser & Vastukar.)
Gita Press Pustak Bhandar
Bhiwani- 127021- India
Ph.: 91-01664-42208, 41680

1

Mind and Disease

Are you happy, prosperous yet worried ? As a matter of fact worry is the main cause of 2/3 of our diseases. It is an established fact that roots of such diseases precipitate in our mind, whereas symptoms appear in our body. If we assess ourselves, we would come to know about our problems/diseases. During assessment we should recognise our bad habits, narrow thinking and ill feelings, which lead us to such problems.

Whatever we think, we do, whatever we eat, so we think. We are attracted towards identical thoughts and circumstances, for instance we make friends having similar thoughts.

Most of our diseases are nothing, but a result of our mental deformation. We think about the incidents up to a certain level. The diseases might be minor in nature but we make it incurable due to tension.

Emotions like jealousy, hatred or anger, sooner or later effect us in the form of some diesease.

Most of the patients suffering from incurable dieseases say that they had never done any evil and have remained vegetarian and thiest, yet they have been suffering ? Infact, the main cause of their problems is tension, for instance, a person could see things clearly for only 5 to 10 minutes after waking and thereafter darkness would appear before his eyes. He was taken to various eye specialists but it was of no avail. Finally he was asked about his mental and emotional problems. After repeated persuation he narrated the unruly acts of his mother and how she had destroyed his happy family.

Since then he neither wanted to see his mother nor hear anything from her. This suppressed grief and anger resulted in his temporary loss of vision. Psychotherapy relieved his ailment.

In another case, a lady was suffering from rheumatic fever. Her only son, whom she loved dearly was wicked and cruel towards her. All her dreams and aspirations crashed, she became depressed and ill. As no amount of treatment helped her, she was advised to meditate and as a result her complaints gradually disappeared.

If flowing river water was obstructed, it gradually takes the shape of a flood, breaking every barrier, creating havoc around. Similarly if feelings are suppressed they create an invisible uproar resulting in mental disbalance.

It is harmful to express something before someone out of emotion, but their suppression leads to tension. There are three ways to prevent this:

(a) Laugh or cry in plenty.
(b) Put forth your problems before a capable guide so that he can guide you on what is right and what is wrong, to vent ones emotions for progress and health.
(c) Feelings may be expressed in some other ways.

People generally supress their passions which results in mental diseases like conflicts, frustrations, etc. In a state of intense emotions, the posionous chemicals produced in our body, may become dangerous for our sanity unless shed through the eyes.

Infact, disease is caused by suppression of emotions which creates a disturbance in the physical functioning of the body and thus the person becomes diseased.

Thus to remain healthy, accept every issue innately and without tension. For e.g.:- frustrated people are generally prone to cancer. The number of people becoming cancer patients due to polluted feelings is more than those who smoke and drink alcohol.

Initially, air, gout, rheumatism, indigestion and change of season were considered to be the main reasons of physical illness, but latest research reveals that mind dominates the entire body. Apart from regular food and walk, it is also essential to mitigate mental pressure and tension.

There are two types of mental passions. The first type includes morality i.e., deception, jealousy, kidnapping, theft, cheating, attack, misconduct, etc. The second type includes joy, worry, apprehension, doubt, sex, disappointment, etc. By observing certain institutions one can avoid tension and evil feelings.

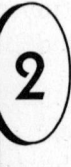

How to be Happy

1. Trust in God :

It is a fact, that once you have faith in God, you don't require anybody. Your life will be filled with joy, hope and merriment.

2. Do not cast stealthy glances in others life :

Casting stealthy glances in other's life is the main reason for disturbing peace at an international level. Instead of taking care of their own homes, ladies keep an eye on other peoples activities around. They try to talk about others as to why they are happy or unhappy. Such stealthy glances develop mental imbalances in our families thereby creating tension, which leads to illness.

3. Do not interfere in other's affairs :

A powerful country or society always wants to dictate a poor country or society. We interfere in other's affairs with the feeling that they are not correct, therefore it is our duty to correct them. In the process we completely forget that God has created us individually and every person is tied up with their own culture. Why should we be disturbed for them ? We may maintain peace if we concentrate on our own work, otherwise we invite unwarranted tension which automatically leads us towards various physical problems.

4. Learn 'forget and forgive' policy :

Our major weakness is that we do forgive but we cannot forget inflicted insults and as such it keeps burning within ourselves. It affects our sleep and comfort, we become hypertensive and develop ulcers. Believe in God's theory of 'Karma', as you sow, so shall you reap'. Life is short so we should not waste it on petty matters.

5. Do not expect undue praise:

Remember everyone is selfish in this world and except for a 'Karmyogi' no one praises you without a selfish motive. If, at some time you have nothing, your own followers will find fault in you and leave you. Work with honesty and zeal, and leave the rest to God.

6. Do not be jealous :

Due to jealousy even the biggest state falls down. In a fit of jealousy for others we forget our objective in life and create tensions for ourselves. We are rewarded or punished on account of our previous birth. The essence of life is to perform your duty honestly, but never be jealous of others.

7. Learn to smile :

Learn the art of similing as it attracts even strangers, whereas a gloomy face causes irritation. A smile doubles your face value. People with this virtue can do more work and also get a lot of work done from others.

8. Learn to bear, what is not in your control :

Sorrow happiness, profit loss, etc. are a part of human life. However some sorrows and losses are caused by nature. Therefore grieving for such sorrows / losses is not thesolution, as people will support you only for some time. Under such situations we should leave everything on God and save ourselves from mental trauma and re-gain self power.

9. Do meditation :

Do mediation daily as it provides mental peace, happiness and activeness in the body. Through meditation, God is achieved, as it provides opportunities for self realisation, contemplation and reflection., However before meditation, " Pranayam" is essential.

10. Do not let the mind get deseperate :

"Desperation" is a word which cannot provide "hope". Darkness will prevail all around and there will be no life. Avoid desperation under all circumstances, be optimistic, it will save you from mental and physical problems. Human life is precious and remember if we do not accept defeat, God will help us.

11. Fulfill your duties :

"Shrimad Bhagwat Gita" is based on " Karma" and everything on earth is related to it. " Karma" means performance of duty without thinking about the result. Even in desperate situations, be courageous. People who believe in luck are basically lazy. All the philosphers, scientists, sants, etc. have achieved their goals through their untiring efforts based on the principle of "Karma".

3. Karma and Yog

Duty or deed prepares the future of a person.

Deeds (Karma):

It is three types:

a) **Prompt deed:** I was thirsty. I took a glass of water and had it. It was a prompt deed

b) **Accumulated deed:** I appeared in an examination, invested money in business, applied for a job, etc; these are all deeds but their result will take some time to come, therefore it is called accumulated deed.

c) **Destiny deed:** It is a deed which we did not perform yet got the result automatically viz., someone leaves a "will" in your name, you receive unknown wealth or without performing any deed got a partnership or a job in a business. It clearly indicates that we are being rewarded / punished on the basis of our accumulated deeds performed during the previous birth.

Therefore if we want to avoid diseases, we should not only take care of our eating habits but also change our emotions. By adopting the 11 tips mentioned in the previous chapter and through contemplation andreflection we may keep ourselves healthy and happy. Remember, you are a distinguished person in the world.

Performance of duty is known as " deed" which may be good or bad.

Duty /deed prepares the future of a person.

"Yog" (Concentration):

"Yog" has been defined in the Gita in a very simple way. Performance of duties in life successfully is called "Yog". Suppose you are a doctor and have examined a patient carefully and charged a reasonable fees from him, it will be treated as "Yog". On the contrary if you did not examine the patient carefully but charged him a huge amount, it will not be treated as "Yog".

Most of the people misunderstand the meaning of "Yog". According to them "Yog" means meditation only which is also essential for physical fitness and if it is performed regularly it may change the life of an individual.

The great Sage Pantjali defined the word "Yog" as "concentration of mind".

Deed Process:

It is of three types:

a) **Purity deed method:** It is based on " I should perform my duty without waiting for a reward". For instance at midnight, you rush to the doctor as your son is not well. You ask him about the fees but the doctor gets ready and says that the fees can be decided later on, let me first perform my duty as a doctor.

b) **Exhibitionist deed method:** According to this method. " I will perform my duty but will not leave my reward". In terms of the above mentioned incident, the doctor will say that he would see the patient, but later on charge Rs. 100/- as fees.

c) **Pre –dominance deed method:** " Unless I do not get the reward in advance, I will not perform my duty". Therefore the pre-dominant doctor will not go with you to examine the patient unless the fees is paid to him in advance.

Now if any person argues that he will not perform any duty and would thereby save himself from doing any good or evil, his thinking would be considered wrong because even the action of eating, drinking, sleeping, awakening, etc. are all parts of a duty. If everyone stops performing their duty and sits down not doing anything, believing in their destiny, the entire human race would vanish from this universe.

A person who believes only in destiny will never perform any duty and would thus lose everything.

If students mainly believe in destiny and do not study properly, they will never achieve success in examination. If you get wealth due to destiny, but are not performing the duties required to utilise the wealth, it will go off. Infact duty is paramount in life and everybody is expected to perform it in the right perspective. The principle, "perform your duty and forget the result" should not be defined in the light of vested interests.

A person is independent in performing duty but is dependent on its result. In other words we are rewarded or punished on the basis of our deeds or misdeeds either in the present life or in the next life (re - birth).

For instance, you have performed your duty by taking a cold drink and ice cream for which you were independent. Subsequently you suffered from cold and loose motions, thereby you become dependent to face all such problems.

Uttering God's name mitigates the worries and also provides strength to face such worries. After examining a patient, doctor issues medicines and also instructs the patient to observe certain preventive measures. However if the preventive measures are not taken, the patient will not recover from his illness. Under the circumstances, it would not be fair to blame the doctor. Infact we may keep ourselves fit and healthy by following the previously mentioned eleven facts and by keeping mental tension away from us. Only then, we may lead a full life.

Pranayam:

In "Pranayam" breathing exercise is carried out to enable the lungs to purify the blood in the body to the maximum and thus, may mitigate the burden on the heart. Through "Pranayam" an unsteady mind becomes stable. Deep breathing means a long life.

Pranayam has four parts: -

a) **Suppliment :** Taking a deep breath gradually is called suppliment.
b) **Antarkumbhak :** Withholding the breathing is called antarkumbhak.
c) **Rechak :** To expel the inhaled air gradually is rechak.
d) **External :** To expel and withhold air is external Pranayam.

Hymn :

The speciality of hymn is mainly based on the selection of words in a specialised manner. They are arranged in accordance to special laws of phonetics.

Recitation of a hymn for a long time provides a peculiar type of energy in the body as well as in the surrounding atmosphere.

The sound of such words creates sound vibrations. Infact an ascetic worships air, which is done through some special methods of Pranayam. Therefore a scholar of "mantras" is not less than any ascetic.

As a matter of fact, the science of 'mantra' is useful in removing physical and mental diseases.

4

Mantra

Mantra worship :

Words have unlimited power. Speech plays a major role in making friends or foes.

Mantra worship is a mysterous method through which mysterous power canbe produced in a large quantity. "Mantra-power" is full of miracles.

Once a small troop of Nepolean's army was marching over a bridge. The bridge fell down and the soldiers were swept away by the river. Later, they realised that the bridge fell down due to the orderly sound of the soldiers foot steps. Since then, a rule has been passed, that the army will not go over a bridge in an orderly manner.

Every one knows about the famous musician Tansen who created miracles by virtue of his music during Akbar's dynesty.

Today, music is not restricted for entertainment only. Rather, scientists have achieved success through music, which is being used for various purposes.

Our feelings and thoughts are associated with mantras and therefore a constant use of "mantra" purify our thoughts and feeling likewise

Importance of mantras depends upon the words chosen. And when the mantra is continuously recited in the same manner for a long period, a special kind of energy is born. By repeatedly reciting a mantra, not only the man's body and mind becomes excited, but simultaneously, the environment in which it is recited also gets provoked by the sound waves which are created by the effective words. Word is a subject of the sky. Thus the sky is workshipped by a person who recites mantras i.e. a mantrik. Yogi's adore air, life power is collected by way of air. In view, mantirks are senior than yogis. A mantrik is not lesser than a yogi.

To get rid of both physical and mental problems, mantras have proved very beneficial.

Mahamritunjaya Mantra :

"Om Haum Jum Sah Om Bhur-Bhuvah Svah

Om Tryambakam Yajamahe, Sugandhim Pusti-vardhanam. Urvarukam-iva, Bandhanan-mrtyor-muksiya mamrtat.

Om Svah Bhuvah Bhuh Om sah jum haum on."

5

Mental Crime

While sitting at the sea shore, watching the waves, sometimes changes ones thoughts and attracts one towards spiritualism. The energy generated from the waves and clamour of the sea, cultivates multiple ideas in the mind of an individual.

As religion is not an issue for argument but faith, similarly some issues are understood through wisdom and not argument. An individuals behaviour and deeds depend on his values and upbringing. Nothing canbe done at a later stage.

People, most of the time think about themselves and their families. The rest of the time they think of others, of which more than 50% of the time they think negatively of them. This is considered as a mental crime.

Harm canbe done to oneself and others. If one smokes, drinks or is an atheist it is a personal harm. However, if we are quarrelsome and fight with others, or we don't keep our surroundings clean, we cause ourselves and others harm, which canbe termed as a mental crime.

No religion or human right commission allows us to commit a mental crime. It is an act of cruelty to ones self as well as towards the family and society. It affects the health and the family adversely.

With a view to avoid negative feelings, one must think 25% about ones self, 25% for family, 25% of religion and 25% of the country and society during moments of leisure.

However being a human being, negative feelings are bound to come naturally. To avoid such situations, people belonging to the thiest category should adore and recite the name of God, whereas and atheist should sing a song, think about his family or read a book because our body may need rest but not the mind.

I do believe that if a person stops committing mental crime, he will get an opportunity to assess himself which will bring elegance in him and would lead him towards salvation.

When we stop thinking about others we will start thinking about ourselves, and then evil automatically goes off.

6 Behaviour

Daily routine behaviour :

Bring a change in your style of talking.

1. Do not use useless and boring words.
2. Use of words through which we try to prove ourselves superior should not be used.
3. Be clear about what ever you talk. It you commit something, keep it up otherwise don't promise. Don't make promises you can't keep.
4. Do not use authentic terms in regard to measurement if it is done by ones estimation only, without actually weighing it.
5. In case measurement is not done by the standard means and is being done individually, in such circumstances, we should not claim for its authenticity. For instance, our claim that the item is 500 gms., maybe wrong as the weight of that item might be a little less or more. Therefore it would be appropriate to say that the weight maybe 500 gms., approximately.

6. Be alert and talk with confidence. Whenever you go out or talk to anybody, be alert and talk with confidence, so that your say carries weight. Here 'alert' means to have patience of hearing and understanding others, only then, you may leave your impression.

7. Do not cast sarcastic remarks. Do not make use of sentences like "why will you recognise me", "you are a big man", etc. as they give a wrong impression to that person. The person concerned will either remain quite or retort in a similar manner. Sometimes a person is lost in his own thoughts, in such a situation you initiate and meet him.

8. Must appreciate where necessary. The great poet Woodsworth has written that a thing or person, if deserves appreciation should be appreciated whole heartedly. But fake appreciation is not good as it will prove you to be a sycophant in the eyes of others. Whereas deserving appreciation will add honour to your personality.

9. Express joy and you must thank the person expressing it. You must express your happiness over a commendable task done by others. When someone is expressing his joy over our success or appreciation, ensure that you extend your thanks to him.

10. Beg pardon for your mistakes. In case someone has pointed out your mistake or you have realised one on your own, don't hide it but beg pardon for it

11. Use of "if you do not mind, may I say one thing". before any bitter truth you have to tell. In this way you can express the truth politely and at the same time it will not hurt the person concerned.

12. Must give clarification. It is essential to clarify your saying. Generally it is seen that we express our views concisely and thus the party concerned does not understand what has been said; as a result one of us may get into an embarrassing position.

13. Remember the name of people, so that you may call them by their names on meeting them for the second time. Remember that a respectful address always pays rich dividends.

14. Make use of these words, 'excuse me', 'please', 'thank you', 'welcome', etc. frequently. In our daily conversation if we make use of the above cited words, it adds another cap to our personality.

    For example- Please be seated,

    Excuse me, I am just coming,

    Thank you for your visit/present.

    You are welcome at our factory, house, shop, etc.

In case we do not use these sentences our personality assessment becomes nil.

15. While going to meet some acquaintance, first of all ask about their well being. When two people meet each other or talk on the telephone, they start beating about the bush, which is wrong. Clarify your purpose of visit or call, but first of all ask about their well being. It makes the relation stronger.

16. Smile and make others smile. The secret of good mental and physical health is smile and making others smile. Keep company of cheerful people. It is not good to be serious all the time as it develops tension. Read humourous books or watch humourous films (if you are not a saint or spiritualist).

17. Remember God is thirsty of feelings and not of worship. It is not necessary to devote two hours for

worship everyday, but to remember God. What is necessary is to worship God for some time and remember him every moment of the day.

18. Take care of others convenience. It is wrong to anticipate that others will take care of our convenience. They may or may not, but we must take care of others convenience where ever we go. If a particular person is not good, leave his company but if it is not possible due to certain reasons, then compromise with the situation and not with the principles.

19. Do not expose anyone forcefully to the extent that he might go away hurt, or say 'no' bluntly. For example:-

   a) Suppose you want to ask for Rs. 1000/- as contribution from a person who is not in a position to give so much. In such a case, do not force him for a donation or he will be bound to say 'no'.

   b) If we know some weaknesses of a person and expose them before others, then the person will not hesitate to break relations with us.

   c) Similarly if we have to get work done from some body who is reluctant, we should not force him.

20. Say 'no' clearly. Due to confusion or misunderstanding, friendships and relations are broken. For instance, if somebody asks for some assistance from you and you are capable of doing so, either say yes or clearly say 'no' to him. Obviously your 'no' will hurt him but at the same time he will regard your principles. On the other hand if you create confusion, and do not give a clear answer, it may hamper relations.

21. Go to meet acquaintances in sorrow. How so ever busy your are, you must pay a visit to acquaintances

in sorrow. In case it is not possible to visit in person, send your representative or talk on the telephone. Such gestures provide relief to the person in distress. Also there must be someone to console grief sticken people.

22. Before lending money think carefully, because if it is not returned in time you would be in an embarrassing situation. Therefore it is advisable to give only such an amount, whose loss is bearable, incase not returned.

23. Be liberal in your views. There is a notion "listen to all, but do what you feel good about", but if someone gives good advise which carries no risk, it should be accepted without making arguments. Remember arguments are not desirable every time.

24. Must compile good books and good people. It is not necessary that good people may help you with money, they could benefit you by virtue of their mind and vision. In the same way, we must read good books for atleast 15 minutes daily dispite our pre-occupancy as it will enrich our knowledge and make us bold and courageous.

25. Do not argue on every issue. Argument means another aspect of an issue which is more relevant than the first. But unnecessary arguments are never considered justified. For example:
    a) If you do not agree with someone, it does not mean your denial. Secondly if a person is putting froth logical aspects, you should keep quite, listen and reflect on it.
    b) Sometimes even a simple advice from a layman canbe fruitful viz., do not read while lying down.

26. Nobody is honest. In the wake of responsibilities and competitions in the present age, nobody is completely honest (leaving exceptions), therefore one should not

Behaviour 21

claim on each and every issue that I always speak the truth. Infact we should not exaggerate about speaking the truth or lie. The best course to express one's self is that, "I am not always truthful but I do not have habit of telling lies".

27. Take care of small issues. We must have a broad mind and a liberal heart as people who get tense on small issues cannot make progress in life.

28. Never be pessimistic. Floating of pessimistic feelings in our mind is human behaviour, therefore in such moments we should divert our attention to reading books or in other modes of entertainment. It is a fact that if we take such feelings in a positive manner, it will give us mental peace.

29. Purchase things within capacity. Cut the cloth according to your need. Do not cultivate the habit of buying things on credit as it not only creates tension of repaying the loan but also affects the future generation adversely.

30. Be careful about time. It is always better to go and meet someone with a prior appointment, however if it is not possible, then be careful about the host's convenience.

    a) Do not visit in the morning because at that time they maybe busy in worship, bathing, exercise, etc. Some people even might be sleeping.

    b) Day time is meant for lunch and a little rest.

    c) At night people have their it own ways to entertain themselves and even family members, if asked to do anything, get annoyed.

Now it is up to the individual to select a suitable time for visiting someone's house.

31. Write down imperceptible feelings. By doing so one can avoid tension. For instance, if you have commit-

ted some mistake or have developed an estranged relation with somebody but could not say anything to him directly, write down your feeling, and send it to the concerned party. By doing so, you will feel relieved.

32. Never curse your fate. "Our luck was bad", "despite belonging to a good family we are hardly earning two meals a day", "we are poor", etc. are some sentences which hinder the path of progress. Despite having money a person may not enjoy it. Rather in his old age, his children enjoy that money.

Infact everybody has a similar luck, what counts the most is "Karma" (action).

33. Ambition is good, but to remain tense for the same is wrong. It is good to be ambitious, but to remain tense for fullfilling the ambition is wrong. Everybody wants to earn wealth but if a person works day and night for the same and involves himself in many jobs all together, it will disturb him mentally, spoil his health and adversely affect his family life.

34. Do not expect much. Never expect much from your family or from known or unknown people as undue expectation leads towards dissatisfaction. If your expectations are within your control, there will be no cause of tension for you even if someone has helped or not and you will remain content. For example:

    a) To visit a shop or office with the hope of getting a discount or job is not good, as it leads to dissatisfaction and disappointment.

    b) We expect our children to support us during our old age, but if it does not happen, we get disappointed.

7
Protection of Babies & Animals

Protect wild creatures and babies in the womb.

God has given wisdom to human beings. Using wisdom in solving problems is the symbol of a successful human being.

There is no doubt that there are many problems in life, but one problem is very important which is generally ignored by us due to our ignorance or ego and that is about the birth of a baby.

Protection of the baby in the womb :

Thinking about abortion on the pretext of (a) price rise (b) keeping age difference between children, etc. is wrong. Human beings are considered civilised, religious and wise, yet they make lame excuses for their own benefit. However, if a baby is conceived and is not desired due to any whim or fancy of the parents, they may go to any extent. Those who do so are cruel. Infact the government is spending huge amounts of money on family planning and if despite taking measures, a child is conceived, it should be accepted as a boon from God.

A 30 minute silent film prepared by America is based on abortion and can be seen along with the family. Through an ultrasound screen, a view of the womb has been portrayed, live, as to what the baby feels in the womb during the process of abortion. It clearly shows how the baby becomes restless when instruments touch him inside the womb and cut the baby into pieces. Although screams of the baby are not heard by anyone yet it is a murder which is done in the womb itself. The view shown in the picture is full of cruelty, heartlessness and helplessness which is enough for human beings to bow their heads with shame. Therefore your cooperation is expected in this cause.

Protection of wild creatures :

All creatures while living in water, earth or sky should be protected as nature has sent them to live in.

Every issue cannot be understood through argument. We should understand and follow certain things on our own discretion. Non-vegetarians may put forth an argument, that if they do not eat it, the population of such animals will increase. If a similar argument is placed before them about man eaters perhaps they will not agree to it.

As I have said earlier it is not an issue of argument but discretion. It is justified for some people to eat flesh and wear leather clothes like, those residing in snowy places e.g. North pole etc. and where there are no crops, but it seems unjustified to eat flesh where everything in available.

Evil cannot be removed from the earth forever but disease canbe eradicated for all, through efforts.

If we stop buying fancy items made of animals to decorate them in our drawing rooms, we may get an adequate quantity of leather for our shoes and footwear. But our demands for fancy items made of crocodile/snake skins are wrong as it would lead to the killing of innocent animals/ reptiles.

We have a cassette titled 'Head and stal' (by Hon'ble Smt. Menaka Gandhi) which shows us how animals are brutally killed by human beings for the purpose of eating and for making fancy items from their skins.

Is it a demand of civilised people or wealth is everything ? Then why are innocent animals being killed by human beings so brutally ?

The best way to save animals is to be purely vegetarian and abandon use of leather items. However, as I mentioned earlier it is difficult to remove evil from the earth completely, similarly all the people on earth may not become vegetarian, but the following suggestions could be adopted:

a) Avoid using items made of leather.
b) Fibre made things are more durable than the leather made items.

Do you know ?

1. Almost in every brand of foreign made toffees, chocolates and chewing gums, an ingredient made from cow's beefbone is mixed.
2. 80% lime (edible) is prepared form oyster shells and before using them, worms inside their bodies are killed.
3. Silver and gold leaves (edible) are manufactured by keeping small pieces of gold and silver on the

intestines of freshly killed animals.
4. Egg contains the embryo of a hen.
5. Almost every shampoo is tested on the eyes of a rabbit who may become blind, before launching them in the market. Therefore only use those shampoos which are not tested on animals.
6. Calf leather is made from calfs skin by throwing a live calf into boiling water.
7. In China, Korea and Vietnam extent of cruelty is seen in their restaurants which offer bloodshed food". *Example:*

   a) Cats are put in a cage for sale on customer's demand. A particular cat is taken out of the cage and put into a boiling water tank. After 10 minutes it's outer skin is removed and sold to the customer for making his favourite dish.

   b) Snakes are tortured by pricking pins in to their mouths, in the process the blood which comes out is collected and used for soup etc.

   c) Monkey kids are electricuted in such a manner that they are neither dead nor alive. Thereafter in the presence of customers their heads are incised and the brain is eaten.

   d) Live, small fishes are put into a bowl with water. The customer then puts some liquor into the bowl and sets it on fire. The small fishes roll about in agony and finally die. These dead fishes are then eaten.

Thoughts of Great Men:

Sh. Richard Bustor said, "Man is the cruelest enemy of himself and others".

According to William Saroyam, " Among all the creatures on this universe, a human being is the biggest liar who claims to be the best."

Shakespeare says, "Even crueliest of all cruel animals is kinder than human beings."

President Lincoln has written, " I do not care about the religion of that person whose dogs and cats condition, is not better than himself."

According to French thinker Mr. Karneez, "Surgical operations carried out for scientific experiments are unbelievable and can safely be termed as heinous acts."

Dr. Jahannes Hale, a kind hearted reformer has written, " It is my confirmed opinion that if people could see surgical operations carried out in science laboratories with their own eyes, they would punish these surgeons without waiting and going to court."

"O! human beings stop killing animals. It is against humanity to kill animals and make use of them for selfish motives. A person who does so should be prepared to meet a similar fate".

— *Phyathegorus*

As you eat so shall be your heart :

In big slaughter houses, animals are cut at an average of per minute and the process of taking out their skins begins immediately, even prior to their becoming lifeless. For getting white flesh, a procedure is adopted in which death takes place gradually.

At the place of killing, animals become hostile, therefore either his eyes are taken out or his tail is broken. In a butcher shop we never taste a piece of mutton, whereas in a vegetable shop we can taste raw vegetables because that is our genuine food. Keep a child, a chicken, a kitten and an apple in a room. You will find that as per the law of nature, the child will go for the apple whereas, the cat would attack the chicken.

- *Arenest kasbee*

Various diseases are developed by eating flesh. Infact we take non-vegetarian food just to keep in good health but we forget that at the cost of health, we invite various, serious diseases.

For instance, a peculiar type of worm which harms the liver is found in middle aged sheep, cow, bull, pig, goat and other animals. When we eat the flesh of these animals, these worms enter our body, as a result we develop hepatitis.

In other words, various types of insects, worms bacteria, viruses, etc. are found in animals and birds, and they enter our bodies when we eat the flesh of such animals or birds. Thereafter we become victims of animal born diseases.

As it has been stated earlier, these diseases have spread all over the world, as flesh is taken in almost every country.

■■

8
Knowledge of Personalities

Experience :

It is essential for a skilled administrater to have knowledge about personalities so that he may alert himself at the time of assigning tasks to the employees.

1. Clever/Skilled People :

   a) On an average, short people are skilled in their behavior and are efficient in getting their work done.
   b) A person who talks with a slanting glance.
   c) A person with a hunch back, one eye and limp. Does not have a neck by birth.
   d) Who make their eyes narrow, slit like, while talking.

2. A Fradulent Person :

   a) Who cannot talk while making an eye to eye contact.

b) People who look above while talking.
c) Whose eyes are narrow, slit like or become like that, while talking.
d) People with a hunch back, one eye, limp and no neck since birth.
e) Who make different contortions of the eye while talking.
f) Who do not raise their eyes while talking.

3. People Who Cannot be Defeated Easily :
a) People with a hunch back, one eye, limp and no neck since birth.

4. Incredible People :
a) A person having a deep mole in his cornea.

5. Treacherous People :
a) Who does not have a neck.
b) Who does not have hair on his chest.

6. Argument Prone Women :
a) Who have hair on their hands and legs.
b) Who have hair all over the body.

7. Eloquent Person :
a) Limp, one eyed or hunch backed since birth.
b) Who does not have hair on his chest.
c) Who has a mole on his cornea.
d) Short people.

8. Subtle Thinker or Conspirator :
a) A reserved person who simply smiles even at a hilarious situation, when everybody is laughing; he just smiles like Socrates or Brutus.

Knowledge of Personalities

9. Obstinate Person :

a) Who's thumb is straight.
b) Who has a wide forefoot.
c) A person with mingled ege brows.

10. Men or women whose date of birth falls on, 10,19,28 are active, impatient, optimistic, self aware, brilliant and egotistical in nature.

11. Men or women whose date of birth falls on 2, 11, 20 29 have a wild imagination, are artistic, moody, sensitive, fickle minded, tolerant, sympathise with others and love nature.

12. Men or women whose date of birth falls on 3,12,21, 30 are sporty, moody, artistic, sacrificing, secretive, confident, dignified, frank and argumentative in nature.

13. Men or women whose date of birth falls on 4,13,22,31 are energetic, revolutionary, active, impatient, optimistic, self aware, brilliant and egoistical nature.

14. Men or women whose whose date of birth falls on 5, 14, 23, are artistic, witty, methodical, mentally energetic, shrewd, intutive, diplomatic, curious, quarralsome, fault finders, have a narrow outlook and restless nature.

15. Men or women whose date of birth falls on 6,15,24 are lovable, sympathetic, adorable, diplomatic, selfish, careful, balanced, have a changeable mood and self indulgent in nature.

16. Men or women whose date of birth falls on 7, 16,25 are original, restless, independent, diplomatic suspicious, ambitious, resevered, intutive, selfish, have a great imagination, are artistic, moody, sensitive, fickle minded, tolerant, sympathetic and lovable in nature.

17. Men or women whose date of birth falls on 8,17,26 are ambitious, hardworking, practical, honest, insistent, creative, changing, suspicious, rebelious, truth seekers, dutiful, gloomy and unconventional in nature.

18. Men or women whose date of birth falls on 9,18,27 are dashing, aggressive, courageous, resistant, impatient, violent, active, enterprising, pioneering, turbulent, torrid, intense, shrewd, energetic, determined and independent in nature.

■ ■

9

Invaluable Knowledge

1. If any action hurts or creates a misunderstanding, even if it is for the betterment of the present or future, should be abandoned.

2. Do not leave the company of noble people.

3. Do not ask the fare directly from a taxi, rickshaw or tempo driver for reaching your destination in a new place. It would be advisable to visit some shopkeeper nearby. You can get correct information about the place as well as the amount of fare to be paid.

4. Always buy T.V., V.C.R, refrigerator etc., from local shopkeepers, even if the prices are not satisfactory. It will save money and time incase any defect is detected in those items during the guarantee period. They can then be easily replaced or repaired.

5. Make it a habit to save money regularly as it is the best and easy way to overcome financial hardships.

6. Whenever you think of starting some business do not ground it on the pretext that funds are not

sufficient. A small capital is a boon and not a curse as it activates your mind to earn more.

7. Keep learning the art of saving money even if the salary is less, if you learn this art, you will not face a financial crisis ever.

8. Do not buy cheap and low quality items. Always go for standardised, quality items.

9. Keep yourself informed about the educational progress of your children and make laison with the school teachers in this regard.

10. Encourage your children to purchase books and establish a library. Also present good books to your children every year and enhance the number and quality of library books.

11. Whatever the children are selling, you must buy something to encourage them.

12. After giving a disciplinary punishment to the children, learn the art of talking to them with a smile.

13. After assigning any task to the children, ensure that the task has been understood by them properly. By adopting this procedure, you will be able to get the work done correctly.

14. Develop the habit of saving and utilising money in your children from childhood, and discourage them from depending on others.

15. You must read out good moral stories to the children, as they will help them throughout their life.

16. Efforts must be made to remove fear from the timid children. Encourage them to become courageous.

17. Advise children not to indulge in any wrong,

difficult or daring tasks on the instigation of any friend or person.

18. Do not keep anything except toys within the reach of babies and small children.

19. Invariably attempt easy questions in an examination first.

20. Instruct children not to respond to any unknown person. Neither should they take anything from him nor go alone to an unknown place, with him.

21. Do not drive the vehicle at a high speed, particularly after getting allured by children.

22. As per requirement, assist your wife in her household chores and also ask children to help her.

23. Always keep a list of household items in your pocket and bring those items on your way home.

24. Whenever the national anthem is sung, pay respect to it by standing up in your place.

25. Success in life depends upon, qualification, courage. Don't an oppertunity, it knocks only once.

26. Life does not depend on what happened with you but on what you learn from such situations.

27. Before lending a big amount to anybody find out about that man from other people with whom he has such dealings and after satisfying yourself completely enter into such a transaction.

28. If you want to get information about an unknown person ask the name and addresses of his intimate acquaintances from whom you can collect the required information.

29. Learn the art of decorating rooms methodically.

30. Prepare special food once a week and regularly change the menu. This will help family members from getting bored of eating similar food.

31. Do not leave the kitchen when something is boiling on the gas stove.

32. Do not carry costly ornaments while travelling.

33. Learn the art of preparing different types of receipes.

34. Treat your employees as your own family members and give them similar treatment and honour. In this way, you may retain them for a longer period.

35. Before sharing your secret with others, think twice.

36. Remember, friendship should not be broken over small disputes.

37. The time devoted for establishing a friendship between two people is not a waste and this aspect should be remembered.

38. Be careful while making a monetary transaction with friends, or you may lose both.

39. Do not exhibit carelessness towards the job assigned to you. Make it a habit to complete the task. This will save you from embrassing situations with your employer.

40. Do not leave the present job unless and until you are sure of getting another job.

41. Do not work with people or in companies whose character or reputation is in doubt.

42. If you are not satisfied with your present job, you may leave it and get another job. But do not criticise your employer on the grounds that he is responsible for your disontentment.

Invaluable Knowledge

43. Lead your life in such a manner that whenever people talk about kindness, compassion and greatness, they must talk of you as well.

44. Prepare your will and register it in the Registrars office in time.

45. However occupied you maybe in your life you must spare some time for religious books, be it the Gita, Bible or Kuran, you must go through these books.

46. Do not allow pesimistic feelings, if they disturb you, think of those who are weaker or less priveleged than you. It will automatically bring you back to normal.

47. Do not exchange articles with your friends without any reason.

48. Do not mixup with scrounderels or people with a doubtful character.

49. Do not hesitate to purchase good books as books are a man's best friend.

50. Do not forget to touch parents feet daily.

51. Restrict your attention on improving things rather than buying a huge quantity of things.

52. You must maintain some fundamental feelings and don't care for others who criticise your feelings.

53. Always honour good thoughts and ideas. Do not discard them simply because somebody tells you to.

54. Always adopt methods for earning money which satisfy your soul and mind and then increase your bank balance.

55. Be competent to mould yourself according to circumstances.

56. Do not purchase edible items when you are hungry as you might buy items in an excess.

57. Do not try to break relations which cannot be tied later.

58. Do not get disturbed in difficult times as it is a part of life. Try to overcome such difficulties through sheer courage and patience.

59. Sometimes thrilling moments come in one's life and such moment must be utilised.

60. Always extend sympathy towards those who really deserve it.

61. Never give a wrong advice to anyone.

62. Never lead a life with a parochial vision, always have a colossal vision.

63. Sometimes speaking the truth becomes harmful to self or others. Therefore after assessing the situation avoid telling the truth to a certain extent, if you feel the truth might harm others or self.

64. Do not indulge in back biting of others.

65. Neither see violent films yourself nor let your children see them. Do not buy items from parties who sponser programmes with a view to ruin our future generation.

66. Money cannot bring happiness in your life.

67. Do not sell your soul for the sake of getting money, power, post or fame.

68. Do not be careless about paying tax. Pay your tax in time and maintain a separate file for that purpose, so that papers canbe located when required.

69. Always contribute something to people raising funds for a good cause.

70. Casting a vote is your right, therefore exercise this right.

71. Get business or education advice from professionals &not form non-professionals.

72. On becoming old, do not remain inactive as it will adversely affect your body. Make a habit to go out for a walk daily.

73. Do not initiate a break in social relations, customs and traditions.

74. Make a habit to re-fill petrol or diesel in your vehicle when is reaches it's reserve level.

75. Before going for sight-seeing, you must read about those places in advance.

76. Before going on a railway or air journey, enquire by telephone whether the train or flight is on time.

77. Develop the power of taking decisions and improve your modus operandi of taking decisions.

78. Make a habit to drink atleast two liters of water daily.

79. Virtue and vice are generally found in every person. Therefore always try to adopt virtues and not vices.

80. Display your residential address at a place from where even a new person can locate your house, without difficulty.

81. Customs have their own religious importance, therefore always respect customs.

82. Never forget to lock your vehicle even if it is parked in your own drive way.

83. Make it a point that 2/3rd of your success in life exclusively depends upon your behaviour with others.

84. Carefully listen and try to adopt good things in your life as it enhances opportunities in life.

85. Whenever you borrow a vehicle for a drive from someone, ensure that you refill an adequate quantity of oil in it.

86. People should be assessed on the basis of their kind heartedness and not by the wealth they have.

87. Learn to live by becoming trustworthy to people.

88. You may advise people but don't expect that it will be accepted and adopted by them.

89. For the purpose of self defence, inveriably keep a stick or an iron rod under your bed.

90. Keep yourself away from various types of litigation cases as it is nothing but wastage of time and wealth. Besides, it causes mental tension.

91. If someone tries to go ahead by pulling you from the back, (on the road or street) let him go.

92. The reason behind any costly item may be due to the high cost of material used in manufacturing that item.

93. Enquire of your beloved ones properly and regularly.

94. Always promise people of giving good items and try to fulfill them too.

95. Never hesitage to praise and congratulate a person who is wearing a new dress.

96. Never show a gloomy appearance, always smile and where ever you go, go with confidence.

97. Always have high intentions.

98. Never compromise with your honesty and ethics.

99. Always keep a notebook and pencil at your bed side as ideas may float in your mind any time at night.

100. Do not hesitate while talking to ladies. Talk with them in a graceful and dignified manner.

101. Never exhibit your ambitions to people as you may become a source of jealousy in the eyes of others and thus you might not be able to achieve your aim.

102. Do not get irritated with others. Live according to your own status.

103. Make it a habit to return borrowed items as per the commitment.

104. Do not beat around the bush, speak in a straight, simple way.

105. Save money for purchasing an item of your choice and buy on cash. It is an ideal habit, develop and maintain it throughout life.

106. Keep smiling always.

107. Despite hard efforts, if you don't get the expected success, be content with whatever you have.

108. Be an open hearted person and also develop a hobby to visit new places now and then.

109. Remember that luck favours only those who put forth consistent efforts through hard work.

110. Do not ignore small opportunities till your ambition in life is fulfilled.

111. Set some principles in life, as the society gives importance to an individual only on the basis of one's behaviour and principles.

112. Never make fake promises.

113. Keep yourself away from casting sarcastic remarks on others.

114. Do not get discouraged if people criticise your work.

115. Try to forget bitter words spoken by people, at the earliest.

116. Pray to God atleast once everyday as it provides mental peace besides, strength at the hour of grief.

117. Before going to bed at night, think about the assignments to be done tomorrow.

118. Before going to the toilet in a new place, check whether water is running or not.

119. To make a married life happy, give attention to your techniques, however small they may be and keep on improving them. By doing so you will be able to lead a happy married life.

120. Do not be dry all the time, learn the art of being romantic.

121. In business, fix up your profit percentage.

122. Always maintain quality and control in business even if your items are a little costly in the market. This way you will maintain your reputation in the market.

123. Make payments on time. If, due to some reason, it is delayed, apologise or if you are unable to pay the whole amount all together, then offer to pay it in monthly instalments.

124. Being hopeful is not bad but to have hopes that the result of the work done will always be in your favour is sufficient enough to disturb your mind.

125. If you go out anywhere take the addresses of known ones and relatives. Try to meet them, as this, not only strengthens old relations but also creates new relations.

126. In government offices, send written letters for the work you want to get done and always keep a duplicate of that letter, get that signed too. Sometimes people you trust might ditch you or leave you when luck does not favor you. In such a case, if you have written documents, the judgement will be in your favour.

10. Relations

If we talk about 'love', we will come to know that love is everything and nothing is possible without love. Even after we leave this world people will continue to remember and love us for our values. But have we ever thought of how much we love our relatives, acquintances, friends, etc. in our daily life ?

If relations with friends or relatives are tense or broken, then we start blaming others. But if we take care of the following things, we may assess ourselves better :

1. Ignore a weak person.
2. Borrowing.
3. Interference in others domestic affairs.
4. Frequent visits.
5. To keep owns say as supreme.
6. Proud for wealth/power.
7. Always blow ones own trumpet.
8. Unable to remove any kind of doubt.

9. Un-due expectations.
10. Meeting with selfish motives.
11. Find faults in others.
12. Maintenance reservance.
13. Making incoherent relations/ friends.
14. Backbiting of others.
15. To be mannerless.
16. To take help from a fraudulent person.
17. To pass sarcastic remarks on each and every issue.

11 Tension

Tension test :

It is true that you do not have control over certain things viz., like price rise, sudden war, natural calamity, iliness, accident, sudden incident, etc. Generally, sorrow and fear jointly aggravate tension but such situations can easily be over come by maintaining patience and if it is not maintained then it adversely affects us, resulting in illness or some other problem.

To have determination, to think about near and dear ones, to take care of small things, to work in an order, to maintain dignity of religion, law and society are virtues of a good citizen. However if we undertake such things under pressure, we obviously invite tension.

Answer the following 60 questions. Each question carries 10 marks, therefore the total marks are 600. If 12 questions are applicable in someone's case, it means, out of 600 marks he gets 120 marks and his percentage comes to 20 %. It indicates that the person concerned is under tension by 20 %, but if care is not taken tension might increase.

1. Dispute in the family.
2. Quarrel with an acquaintance.
3. Divorce.
4. Infertility.
5. Not blessed with a son.
6. Death of a beloved one.
7. Emotional stroke.
8. Illness/accident (of self or some dear one)
9. Not getting the desired item/person.
10. Unemployment.
11. Disturbance in the office.
12. Seperation of children in divorce.
13. After divorce, search for a partner.
14. Unable to carry on business.
15. Loss in business.
16. At the verge of retirement, future apprehensions.
17. Irregular menstrual period.
18. Unresponsive attitude of the partner during sex.
19. Partner's more demand for sex.
20. Difference in likings/recognition with the partner.
21. Seperation.
22. Lack of moral culture / wisdom in children.
23. Marriage- problems of children.
24. Mistakes or lapses committed by children.
25. To make a change in the work style.
26. Apprehensions on exposure of secrets.
27. Family disputes.
28. Worry for career.

29. To mould oneself in a new environment.
30. Worries pertaining to a daughter in law/married daughter.
31. Pressure from seniors during service.
32. Pressure from big businessmen in business.
33. In distress.
34. Borrowing/ lending money.
35. Heartening of ego.
36. Own principles being suppressed by others.
37. Happening of unexpected things.
38. Non-coordination between new and old generation.
39. Neighbours.
40. Helplessness of any type.
41. Dispute of partner with in laws.
42. Frustration.
43. Wish to earn more.
44. To be more emotional.
45. Tension in regard to petty things.
46. Worry to meet new people, place or thing.
47. Transfer.
48. Problems of pregnancy, getting tense regarding the sex of child.
49. In case of repeated miscarriages.
50. Whether husband, wife or children have taken a meal or not, are alright or not, etc.
51. Whether gas, light, door, lock, utensils have been attended to, checked or not.
52. Law, society, religion, communalism, hooliganism, quarrels, tax, etc.
53. If I become so or commit so.
54. Unnecessary tension from anticipating a fear of crowd, height or high speed.

55. Worry due to fear of anticipatory failure.
56. Despite having good health, tension to have good health forever.
57. Tension with regard to family or things.
58. Baseless fear.
59. Keeps burning in remorse throughout life.
60. Not getting promotion whereas companions have achieved it.

12

Dhyan and Yoga

Dhyan and Yoga do not cause any hinderance in the faith or religion of others. Yoga brings prosperity to life and gives the power to endure. One gets liberated from hidden sorrows and fears of the unconscious mind.

Accumulation of carbondioxide occurs during sleep. By practicing 'Dhyan', concentration of oxygen and carbondioxide remains equal. Adernal glands produce adrenaline in stress, fear and calamity. It suspends the digestive system and stimulates the nervous system and heart. It causes vasoconstriction and acts as a brohcnodilator. If stress continues for a long time, the nervous system also gets stimulated, resulting in tension with symptoms like: biting of nails, tossing legs, etc. Such symptom herald or preceed the onset of diseases like diabetes, gastric ulcers, hypertension, cancer, rheumatism, etc. One cannot have a good sleep in excessive stress, he becomes a patient of insomnia. The only remedy to check these diseases is to give complete relaxation to the mind and body. The loss caused by stress cannot be compensated by sleep alone. The body and mind requires maximum relaxation.

The septal region in the head reduces our emotional reactions and lessens or removes tension. We can keep the septal region in a proper state of functioning by 'Dhyan' and 'Yoga'. Mind is the root cause of many diseases and it enhances the effects of diseases. By taking the help of 'Dhyan' and 'Yoga', we can keep our mind healthy. A healthy mind resides in a healthy body. Our entire life is based on breathing. If we practice 'Pranayam' and 'Dhyan' for 10 minutes, it has a direct effect on our body and it enhances our power and vital energy. There are 6000 alveoli in the lungs. Oxygen reaches only 2000 of these when we breathe in the ordinary manner. The remaining 4000 alveoli contain carbondioxide which causes various diseases. A ten minute practice of Pranayam fills these 6000 alveoli with oxygen after removing carbondioxide (CO_2). Consequently, the mind and brain become pure and the body beautiful. You may practice 'Dhyan' for 10 minutes, but practice Pranayam just before 'Dhyan' and before Pranayam do the exercise Bhastrika.

Bhastrika :

We inhale and exhale completely and quickly. The speed of breathing is like that of a blacksmith blowing his bellows. According to the pharmacopia it has the strength to cure 20 types of coughs and respiratory diseases.

Procedure :

(a) Sit erect in Padmasana. Thereafter close one nostril with the middle and ring finger and the other with the thumb.

(b) First remove the thumb and inhale completely and quickly so that your stomach swells up fully. Then close the nostril immediately with the thumb by pressing it.

(c) Remove fingers from the other nostril and exhale completely, so that your stomach is squeezed and then at once close the nostril with the fingers.

(d) Drawing in air through one of the nostril while the other is closed is called Purak and to expel the inhaled air is called Rechak.

(e) Keep your mouth closed throughout.

The nostril from which we practice Rechak, we immediately perform Purak from the same nostril. Then after closing it, we do Rechak and then Purak from the other nostril. This procedure has to be done very quickly and continuously. Do not stop for a single minute also. In 2-3 minutes, breathing becomes heavy the chest will swell up like a balloon and we have palpitations. This is when all the alveoli in the lungs start opening and they will remain open if it is practiced daily. We must exercise Bhastrika after 'Jalneti' so that in case any water remains in the nose, it may come out or dry up. It must be performed before sitting for Pranayam. After Bhastrika put 2 drops of ghee or butter in each nostril so that the skin may remain soft and no irritation occurs. If you sweat or feel unconscious, it means that you have not exercised Bhastrika properly.

Pranayam :

There are four stages of Pranayam. First sit in Padmasana.

(a) **Purak:** Inhale deeply and gradually, upto the count of 5.

(b) **Antrank Kumbhak:** Hold the breath, counting upto 10.

(c) **Rechak:** Exhale slowly counting upto 5.

(d) **Bahirang Kumbhak:** After exhaling, we again hold the breath upto the count of 10.

If holding the breath is difficult, close both the nostrils with the thumb and fingers as in Bhastrika. You can increase the counting period with practice. In the first week 5-10-5-10, in the next week 10-20-10-20 for Purak, Antrang Kumbhak, Rechak and Baring Kumbhak. After Pranayam, practise 'Dhyan'. You will be happy, relaxed and lofty.

Pranayam is a very efficacious exercise to avoid vaginal infection and discharge from the vagina. For this, a women has to do the additional exercise of harmonising the vaginal muscle while doing Purak, contract the vaginal muscles slowly and while doing Kumbhak, keep the muscles in a contracted position. In Rechak, while exhaling gradually, let the vaginal muscles loose also gradually. Do not contract or loosen the muscles hastily. This can only be perfected by practice.

If you can devote 20-30 minutes to your body daily, your body will be obliged. This canbe appreciated well in middle or old age or otherwise all the others will be enjoying themselves and you will be cursing yourselves because your body is ill and powerless. Everyone will be eating sweets, but you will be staring at them as you have a diabetes. Everyone will be eating chaats and pakoras but you cannot, as you are suffering from hypertension. When everyone dances you wont be able to, as you have rheumatism.

The fact is that you laughed when your body was begging for your welfare as you were busy in your enjoyment and earning wealth. Now you have everything but you can't enjoy or use that wealth as you are ill, incompetent (powerless), under stress, and dependant on doctors. You weep but your body langhs.

In the modern era, medical scientists have achieved full knowledge of blood, bones, nervous system, muscles, etc., but cannot claim full control over the complicated structure of the body bestowed by God and nature. This is because an animating force dwells in this physical body which cannot be percieved by modern instruments or machines, nor can one perform surgery over it. Hence, Yogic procedures, Mudras, Pranayam, Dhyan, Yoga are used and these are called Yogic techniques.

Do not use force in Yogic techniques. Yogic techniques and Yogasana are related to the respiratory system and concentration of mind. They, after providing energy and power, establish harmony in the mind and body.

Yogasana are practiced on an empty stomach. Urine and stool should be excreted. Don't use undue strain in an asana because they may cause harm instead. There are many asanas which may harm a person who is suffering from serious diseases like hypertension, asthma, rheumatism, etc. or those who have weak or old bones. Therefore learn the asanas from an expert Yogi and understand their implication.

I am describing some asanas which canbe exercised by every person and are useful in all diseases.

Special Precautions :

1. Do not practice asanas with undue stress or force.
2. Do not practice asanas exceeding one minute, do far less than a minute.
3. Each asana should also be done in the opposite direction, once on the left side, then on the right side.
4. After each asana you must do a Shavasana.
5. All asanas need not be done on the same day. Divide them through out the week or fortnight, or do the

asanas which are useful to you according to your liking and convenience.
6. If you cannot follow an asana by simply reading, contact a Yoga teacher.
7. Old weak people suffering from incurable diseases should not perform asanas.

Surya Namaskar :

If we perform a certain mudra, Pranayam and Surya Namaskar, then we need not practise any other exercise. There are five steps in Surya Namaskar.

First you stand erect and lift both your hands. Thereafter, keeping both legs straight, bend your waist so much that both the hands touch your feet. Now take the position of an animal with four legs. Keep the legs back ward. With the help of both your hands. Bring out your chest like the spreading head of a snake, look upwards, raising the body from the waist upwards.

Do not stand at once. Gradually stand up, going in the manner reverse to the method by which you have completed the asana.

Shavasana (Corpse Pose)

Lie flat on your back like a corpse. Relax all the muscles of the body. Inhale and exhale completely, but slowly.

Sarvangasana

It prevents premature hardening of bones or ossification, cough and constipation. In all, this asana and Halasana are the best and the simplest for the body.

Procedure – Lie down on a carpet, on your back. With the help of both the hands. Lift your hips, slowly.

Lift your legs off the ground and while balancing your legs straight, raise both the legs upwards, towards the sky at a 90° angle. Your hands are pressing against the sides of the back for support.

Halasana (Plough Pose)

It is useful for the spine, digestive power and brain.

Procedure – Its two third procedure is like that of Sarvangasana. Do Sarvangasana, without bending the knees, raise the hips higher and brings the legs over the head till the toes touch the ground. In this asana the waist is completely curved.

Tolasana

It gives power to the palm, wrist, arm and stomach.

Procedure – Take the pose of Padmasana in a manner that the soles are over the thighs. Thereafter place both the hands and palms firmly on the ground and lift your body above the ground as much as you can. Start tossing your body, to and fro in air, slowly.

Kandha Baju Angulian Sakti Vardhak

Arms, shoulders and fingers become powerful and it removes all kinds of defects in them.

Procedure – Stand erect with legs straight, take both the hands backward, breathing deeply. Turn the waist backward; head should also be bent backwards (as far as possible). After bending the back, hold your breath i.e. practise Kumbhak. Stay in that position for a while, and then come forward while inhaling slowly.

Shambhvi Mudra

It is also called Shivbhangima. In this mudra, vision is to be kept on the mediterranean i.e. where the two eye-brows meet. This is the location of Shivji's third eye.

Agochri Mudra (Agyut Bhanyima)

Sit in Padmasana position. If you are unable to sit in this position, sit cross legged in an ordinary way, keeping the waist and head straight.

Concentrate the eyes on top of your nose. Do not put undue strain on the eyes, increase the period of exercise gradually. If the eyes feel stressed, stop it. Exercise both the mudras together as they are the two sides of a coin.

Advantages : it helps in concentration and reduces mental stress and anger. It sharpens the eye sight.

Mukh shakti Vardhak Asana (Mouth Stimulant)

It gives relief in pyorrhea and pimples. It glorifies the face. It helps in killing the bacteria in the mouth.

Procedure – Method is like Pranayam, but we do not breath from the nostrils. Breath from between the lips purse the lips, like a beak, while drawing in the breath, it will make a whistling sound. Close the nostrils with the help of the thumb and fingers. Thereafter close the mouth and swell your cheeks. Perform Kumbhak. There will be full pressure on the cheeks. Exhale slowly in Rechak, by making a small, hole like opening between the lips. Repeat 5 times at least.

Blowing a conch (shankh) twice or thrice a day acts as a mouth stimulant. This asana kills those bacteria in the body also, which cannot be removed by any other therapy.

Itkat Asana

It makes the thighs, ankles and waist stronger.

Procedure – Stand erect, keep the legs, 2-3 feet apart, by jumping. Thereafter, bend your knees and lift your arms in a straight manner as in over the head and fold them as in Namaste.

Garud Asana

It gives strength to the ankles and arms.

Procedure – Stand straight. First, rotate or turn the right leg over the left leg in such a manner that fingers of left leg rest on the calf of the right leg.

Utithitha Trikon Asana

It gives strength to the legs, knees, ankles and hands. Also widen the chest.

Procedure – Stand erect, keep the legs 2-3 feet apart after jumping. Thereafter bend one of the legs at the knee joint and lift it in such a manner that the hand of the same side holds the paw of the foot. Lift the other hand straight upward. Face should be on the side of upward hand. The hands or legs should not bend. Also practice on reverse side.

Vir Bhadra Asana

It is useful for the chest and lungs. It gives strength to the back muscles, side muscles and shoulders.

Procedure – Stand erect. Thereafter, bend one leg at the knee joint, take the other leg back to the maximum extent. Turn and curve the chest backwards, lift both hands, folded in a Namaste upwards. Repeat the exercise in the reverse position with the other leg.

You can spread your hand like the wings of a bird also.

Varachhasana

It strengthens the legs and arms. Is helpful in maintaining balance and concentration.

Procedure – Stand erect and bend your right leg and keep it's sole at the root of the left thigh. Keep hands on the waist. Thereafter, lift the hand straight above the head in Namaste mudra. Repeat with other leg.

Suptavajra Asana

It removes tiredness, while giving strength to the muscles of feet and shoulders. It is good for the stomach and brain.

After doing this asana, practise Vajra asana.

Procedure – Sit and bend both your legs backward (like when we pray to God).

Thereafter, take your body backwards so that your head touches the ground. Keep hands backwards or alongside the legs.

Vajara Asana

It gives strength to the entire leg from the hips to the toes.

Procedure – Sit as in Supta Vajara asana. Pray to God for food, health and pure thinking for a few seconds. Thereafter, while sitting, bend your waist forward to the maximum so that the head touches the ground. The hands will remain in front.

Paschimottan Asana

It gives strength to the thighs and keeps the stomach in order.

Procedure – While sitting, keep your legs and knees flat, and waist straight. Bend forward and clasp the big toe of the right leg with the right hand and the toe of the left leg with the left hand. Bring down your head so that it touches the knees. Do not raise your knee to achieve this. Do not use force. Heart patients should not practice this asana.

Dhanur Asana (Bow Pose)

It is the best asana for the legs, stomach and waist. After doing this asana, exercise the Paschimottan asana. (Note: Shavasan should be done after every asana).

Procedure – Lie flat on your stomach, bend the legs backward and upwards over the thighs. Catch hold of each paw with your hands. Then pull both the legs with your hands. Pull the legs towards the head, as much as possible, drawing the chest upwards, off the ground, taking the waist behind. The head should be facing upwards. This is called the Dhanur asana.

■■

Indian Ayurvedic Massage

The technique of massage is in use all over the world since old times. In Unan, this technique was so much in use that when a warrior used to return from the field, full arrangements were made for his massage, slaves were especially kept this purpose.

Julius Ceaser, who was suffering from a nervous breakdown was massaged with a special technique. In India, massage is a part of Ayurveda. In this technique medicines are not taken orally but it keeps the bile, wind and phelgm (Vata, Pitta and Kapha) in balance. Indian sages have written a complete code in relation to the technique of massage as to where and when, which oil or mixed oil is to be used.

A massage functions in two ways on our body :

1. Physical: Massage creates an energy by which blood movement is enhanced.
2. Mental: Touch and rubbing has a magnetic effect on our body and the nervous system gets energised.

It helps us feeling more relaxed. Can induce sleep also.

In the absence of a masseur, one can do self massage, but it is less advantageous. In case of a married couple, they can massage each other if no masseur is available.

The practice of getting a massage from the opposite sex is prevalent amongst the royalty and the rich since the middle ages till today. At that time, male and female masseurs used to be healthy and beautiful. As mentioned earlier, one enjoys it physically and mentally, and this is equally shared by the masseur.

The word massage is derived form the Greek word 'mass' which means to press the muscles by hand and to rub the joints. Since a massage energises the body, care must be taken to conserve this energy. Avoid hard physical or mental labour after a massage, otherwise it will have no value in the real sense.

As a rule, if an experienced masseur, in a good state of mind massages, the patient will recover faster as his emotions and power will be converted into positive energy, which is absorbed by the body of the patient during the massage.

People who are unable to get a daily massage on account of physical problems or business, are advised to get massaged atleast once a week. However a regular exercise is also beneficial as it improves the blood circulation in the body.

Technique of Massage : A massage should be started the middle of the chest. Drench 2-3 fingers in oil, massage slowly, in the upward clockwise direction for one minute and in the anti-clockwise direction for another minute. Thereafter, massage should be done around the navel in the same way for 2 minutes. Then start massaging from the legs or head. The direction of massage on any part of the body, should always be clockwise, anticlockwise, upward and downward.

Another point to be kept in mind while massaging is that no force should be used, rather, the force should be on emotions. Remember if a massage is being done with full emotions, then the emotion in the shape of positive energy will cure the patient. If your emotions are bad, or of a greedy nature then the person will recover late. More time should be given to patients of arthritis and rheumatism.

Rules of Massage :

1. A massage should be performed in a calm atmosphere. Both the patient and the masseur should be patient. They should not talk for best results.
2. Massage should not be done on a cot.
3. Masseur should apply his hand slowly and with reasonable pressure.
4. Massage should be done from below upwards. This improves the blood circulation. In cold massages, it should be form above downwards which helps arteries to work faster.

A blood pressure patient should be massaged slowly from above downwards. It is best to have a massage in the open sun, but when it is intolerable or if there is no sun, it can be performed in a room.

After the massage, take a bath with luke warm water for best results. If you do not wish to bathe, get the body sponged. Before a massage, empty your bowels and take a light breakfast.

People having fever, vomiting, dysentery or swelling should refrain from a massage.

The breast should be pressed gently and massaged slowly in a circular way. It is important to regularly massage the abdomen and thighs of a women who has recently delivered. Never massage the abdomen of a pregnant woman. Don't massage the stomach and thighs during menstruation.

Professionals should use a rubber mat for massaging. Before using it for another patient, clean if with dettol.

A mother is the right person to massage her child. No other person can massage the child as affectionately and wishfully. In case another person massages the baby, it must be done with tender hands. Ghee, butter and almond oil are good oils for a massage. Each and every joint should be massaged in a circular way.

The most important thing for a masseur is that he should perform the massage with all his body and mind. He should concentrate on the part which he is massaging because the energy and emotions from his body, enter the body of the person on whom the massage is being performed.

Personally, I use coconut oil in simple massages if there are no serious or chronic diseases because it is not heavy like mustard, almond or olive oil. Also everyone likes the fragrance of coconut oil. The truth is that each individual has their preference regarding the oil. Coconut oil canbe used all year round whereas mustard oil, almond oil and olive oil cannot be used in summers. In the same way, sandal oil, rose oil etc. are prohibited in winters (except in some particular diseases). Our body absorbs coconut oil easily as it is light and one does not feel greasy after it's use, where as heavy oils have the reverse effect.

Types of Massages :

Indian Ayurvedic massage or swadeshi massage has an important place, and are considered the best in the world.

A massage can be dry, cold, hot or with powder.

Cold Massage : in this technique, a towel is drenched in water. After squeezing, it is rubbed on the body. When it becomes warm it is again drenched in water, squeezed and rubbed. In this procedure, massage is done from above, downwards. Obesity is reduced and arteries become stronger.

Hot-Cold Massage : Two utensils of fresh and hot water are kept. Procedure is same as that of cold water massage, but a hot and cold towel are used alternately. It is good for the nervous system.

Dry and Powder Massage : In this, massage is done by pressing the hands a little harder, gently or by a trembling, tapping pattern of hands. It is done on people who do not like oil or nothing else is available at that time. Generally weak people are massaged with dry hands or with powders, gently.

Electronic Massage : In this process, vibrators are used which have many kinds of attachments e.g. a comb like instrument for the head, sponge like instrument for the face, etc. They create tremors and vibrations and their speed can be controlled.

Massage the soles for a better sleep. Rub oil on the head in the morning for better sight.

Massaging daily or once a week will save us from skin diseases and allergies. It keeps Vata, Pitta and Kapha, i.e. wind, cough and bile in equilibrium. It makes the body beautiful, intelligent and increases confidence.

Massage has always played an importance role in coping up with diseases like insomnia, mental depression, paralysis, polio, obesity, headache, nervous disorders, etc.

Hot oil: Mustard, Olive, Eucalyptus, and Almond oil.

Cold oil: Sandal, Rose, Til oil, etc.

Some important infomation regarding the leading oils.

1. Lettuce oil – Useful in insomnia and disorders of the nervous system.
2. Olive oil – Arthritis, weakness.
3. Sandal oil – Mental disturbances.
4. Almond oil – disorders of the nervous system, brain fag, and old age.
5. Acacia oil- Muscular pain.
6. Fish oil – Weakness, cold, arthritis, joint pains.
7. Coconut oil- Dry hair.
8. Mustard oil- heats the body
9. Sesame/Til oil- used on the head and breasts. Removes sad memories, insomnia, foreign bodes lodged in the body, anxiety and high fever.

The above oils can also be used by mixing each other. Massage children up 3 years for 15-20 minutes, 40-45 minutes on young men, and on old people, as per their consent and health.

While concluding, I wish to convey that if you are massaged once a week, at any time, suiting, your convenience, you will feel the change within a few days itself.

■■

Mudra Therapy

Our body and nature consist of five elements. The basic principle of mudra science is that an imbalance or a disproportionate increase or decrease in any of these five elements causes disease. By balancing and bringing the five elements in proportion, we keep the body healthy. The human body is the best creation of nature and hands are the most important part of it. A peculiar kind of life energy, magnetic waves or aura comes out from the hands. According to acupressure therapy, health lies in our hands. As per the Indian sages, the five fingers represent the five elements, each finger is connected to one element. Modern science also recognises the fact that from each finger tip, different electro-magnetic waves are emitted.

Different fingers represent different elements :

Thumb	-	Fire
Index	-	Air (wind)
Middle finger	-	Sky
Ring finger	-	Earth
Little finger	-	Water

The main curative mudras are as follows :

1. Gyan Mudra,
2. Vayu Mudra,
3. Akash Mudra,
4. Sunya Mudra (Zero Mudra),
5. Pirthvi Mudra,
6. Surya Mudra,
7. Varun Mudra,
8. Jalodar Mudra,
9. Apan Mudra,
10. Pran Mudra
11. Sahaj Shankh Mudra,
12. Apan Vayu Mudra,
13. Ling Mudra,
14. Dhyan Mudra.
15. Shanka Mudra

General Rule for performing Mudras :

1. The above stated mudras are very effective, form the health point of view. Every male, female, young, old, child can do these mudras in any condition and at any time, there is no rule on restriction of time. Mudras like Upasna and Sadhana mudra, canbe performed while walking, sitting, sleeping, travelling in a bus, viewing television, talking, etc., or whenever we desire.

2. A mudra should be performed with both the hands but practicing a mudra with one hand only is also beneficial like in Gyan mudra. Doing a mudra with the left hand affects the corresponding parts of the right side of the body. Consequently, a mudra done by the right hand has an effect on the left side of the body.

3. Apply easy and light pressure while doing a mudra. While performing a mudra, the remaining fingers should be kept straight in a natural way without using force. Touching of two fingers is the most important aspect of mudra. The remaining fingers are kept straight as per convenience.

4. A common man should do these mudras for 10 minutes in the begining. It may be extended to one hour later on, gradually.

5. Some mudras canbe performed whenever and for as long a time as desiered, for example, Pran, Aman and Prthivi mudra. However some like Sunya and Vayu mudra cannot be performed once normal health is achieved as they may prove harmful.

Gyan Mudra

Put light pressure after joining the tips of the index finger and thumb. Pressure is not necessary. Keep others fingers straight in a natural way.

Advantage : Strengthens the brain. Improves capacity and capability to grasp knowledge. Removes ill effects of mental stress. All mental defects and diseases like madness, disturbances, uneasiness, unstableness, anger, laziness, depression confusion, fear, eagerness are cured by doing Gyan mudra regularly. The mind is purified and it becomes peaceful. The face gets an expression of unprecedented delight.

Vayu Mudra

Join the tip of the index finger to the root of the thumb and then press lightly. This is the Vayu Mudra.

Advantage : All kinds of arthritis, joint pains, rheumatism, tremors of hands and legs, sciatica. Colic is also cured by this mudra without any medicine. Patients suffering form these diseases need maximum practice of this mudra.

Akash Mudra

Join the tips of the middle finger and thumb, keeping the other fingers straight in a natural manner.

Advantage : 1. Bone weaknesses are cured by doing this mudra regularly.

2. If stiffness in the jaws occurs while yawning, it will be cured immediately by snapping the middle finger and thumb. This is the reason why many people snap their middle finger and thumb at the time of yawning near the mouth, as though without knowing it's significance.

3. It is useful in heart diseases.

4. Ear diseases which are not cured by Sunya mudra.

Sunya Mudra

Keep the index finger on the 'guddi' (near the tip) of the thumb and then press the middle finger with the upper portion of the thumb, this is the Sunya mudra.

Advantage : It is especially useful in ear diseases. Perform the Sunya Mudra when pain starts in the ear. It will subside within 4-5 minutes. It is also useful in stammering.

Pirthvi Mudra

The tips of the thumb and ring finger are joined in Pirthvi mudra.

Advantage: A weak person gains weight. This mudra should be done by people desiring to put on weight.

It gives vitality. Performing the mudra regularly rejuvenates the body and it remain healthy in all respects.

Surya Mudra

Join the tip of the ring finger to the root of thumb. Press the tip of the ring finger lightly on the thumb. This is known as Surya mudra.

Advantage : It reduces obesity and removes mental stress.

Varun Mudra

Join the tips of the little finger and thumb.

Advantage : 1. Removes dryness of the skin and moisturises it.

2. Purifies blood and increases oily secretions on the body surface.

3. Helpful during lack of water in the blood which causes a stretching sensation and gastric disturbance.

Jalodar Mudra

Keep the little finger at the root of thumb and then press the thumb on the little finger. This is called Jalodar mudra. Other fingers remain straight.

Advantage : It is especially useful, in 'jalodar diseases' and can be performed with Sunya mudra.

Apan Mudra

Join the tips of the middle and ring finger with the tip of the thumb.

In this mudra, the little and index fingers remain naturally straight.

Advantage : 1. The body remains clean and all unwanted liquid and excretions come out easily. Continuous use of this mudra not only enables all the excretions and sweat to come out from the pores of the body but also creates a pious feelings.

2. It controls flatulence and decreases it, as this mudra controls Apaan Vayu.

3. In piles and constipation, this mudra should be exercised regularly for 15 minutes.

4. It also helps in keeping teeth healthy

5. It controls diabetes and defects of the mouth, ear, nose and eyes are naturally cured by it.

Pran Mudra

Join tips of little and middle finger with that of the thumb. Remaining two fingers remain naturally straight.

Advantage : 1. Exercising this mudra daily, increases the power to prevent diseases and makes the vital power stronger.

2. It fills up the deficiency of many vitamins.

3. Physically weak people regain power.

4. Relieves tiredness.

5. Has a good effect on eyes. People desierous of removing all defects and diseases of the eyes should exercise this mudra for 5 minutes daily.

6. Helps Gyan mudra in sleeplessness and Apan mudra in diabetes.

Shankh Mudra (conch)

Keep the thumb of left hand closed in the fist of right hand and join the index fingers of left hand with the right hand thumb. The remaining three fingers of left hand jointly press the closed fingers of the the right hand gently.

Advantage : 1. Performing Sankh mudra for a long time helps in removing all defects of speech. It has a good effect on the throat and thyroid gland, voice becomes sweeter.

2. This mudra has a special relation to the navel.

3. Has a healthy effect on the nerves.

4. Makes the muscular system stronger.

5. It has a very good effect on the digestive system and increases appetite. It sets, the disorders of the intestines and lower abdomen right.

Sahaj Shankh Mudra

It is another kind of mudra where fingers of both the hands are entangled with each other, the palms of both the hands are pressed against each other and both the thumbs are pressed together, parallel to each other.

Advantage : 1. Practice of this mudra cures stammering, lisping and all kinds of voice defects.

2. A singer acquires a more sweeter voice.

3. This mudra has connection with the navel.

4. Has a good effect on internal and external health.

5. The digestive system remains in orders. One digests food quickly and is relieved from gas problems. Provides relief from intestinal and abdominal disorders.

Apan Vayu Mudra

After joining the index finger to the root of the thumb, the tip of the thumb is joined with the tips of the middle and ring fingers. The little finger naturally remains straight.

Advantage : 1. Pain which is not cured by Vayu mudra is cured by the exercise of this mudra.

2. It is a boon for heart patients.
3. Gives immediate relief in headache.
4. Mitigates gas in stomach.
5. Benefits a weak and palpitating heart.

Ling Mudra

Entrap fingers of both hands and keep thumb of either hand, right or left straight.

Advantage : 1. Produces heat in the body, therefore, of special benefit in winters. As long as this mudra is exercised, take maximum water, juice, milk and ghee. If a person is feeling cold due to any reason, it canbe remedied by this mudra immediately. There is a possibility of sweating when exercised for a long duration.

2. As it creates heat in the body, cough is deffused,. Also gives relief in cold, cough and other diseases due to exposure to cold.

Dhyan Mudra

While sitting in 'padmasan', keep the palm of right hand lightly on the palm of left hand. The head, neck and spine should be in a straight position. Eyes and lips should be closed in a natural manner. Concentrate on God or try to remain thoughtless for sometime.

Advantage : One gets mental peace and the brain become stronger. Uncertainty disappears and concentration increases. It creates pious thoughts.

15. Reiki

The word Reiki has been derived from the Japanese language. 'Rei' means 'world wide' and 'ki' means 'life energy', hence, life energy is universal. This energy is power. Energy is the source of all living things, plants, insects, animals and human beings. When the energy exits from the body, he or she is declared dead.

The propounder of Reiki was Dr. Mekau Ushuer of Japan born in the 19th century. He was a Christian scholar and teacher. He got inspiration for Reiki form the writings of Mahatma Buddha. After learning Reiki, he started making disciples and helping people. Amongst his leading disciples were Dr. Hayasi and Mr. Takata.

Reiki is a spiritual and highly naturopathic system of medicine. It was used by Jesus Crist, Guru Nanak, Gautma Buddha and other leading sages. A Reiki master or giver should have the power of high concentration because Reiki is a symbol of truth, generosity and spirituality. Reiki canbe learnt by any child or old person. It has no adverse effects. It cures all mental and physical problems like tuberculosis, cancer, AIDS, asthma, ulcer, sciatica, migraine, weakness, etc. Reiki is a useful therapy for all doctors, psychologist, etc. If Reiki is used simultaneously with other therapies, then it helps cure the sick faster. Reiki helps in liberating bad habits and increases will power, memory, love, spirit and sympathy. It diminishes stress and fear, helps increasing friends and trade and helps avoid all ill designs. It can be used on any tree, plant, animal, house, shop, office, factory, etc. It is a cosmic energy, one gets more and more stronger when he gives Reiki to others.

It is not a religion, hypnotism or tantra, It is a practical truth. As science advances, so does the spiritual world. Either one cannot advance unilaterly.

Ascetics by the power of there devotion blessed people from far or near. The atmosphere where they used to live was very pious and full of love and harmony.

Go to any ashram of a saint, whether he is alive or dead, you will have a feeling of immense peace and serenity. I remember going to the place where Maharishi Arvindo Ghosh was imprisoned, I felt an atmosphere of profound peace and serenity surrounding that room. It is a scientific truth that electrons of the person remain where he lived. If the person has an evil thinking then the particles will have a negative effect. On the contrary if thinking is pure and good, the particles will give a positive result.

These particles remain on earth in the same state as they were and never diminish. A heap of these particles is called energy. These particles remain inside and outside the body.

We are attracted or are compatible with some people, where as with others, we are repelled or are incompatible. This is due to the invisible force or aura. Aura consists of seven colours which are invisible. Whenever a person suffers from a physical illness (acute or chronic) like headache or cancer, energy decreases and the aura is disturbed on account of which problems arise. The spiritual therapy then applied to remedy this is called Reiki. If energy increases it is not good as the man suffers from fever, etc. On the other hand, if energy decreases, then also it is not good. By the application of Reiki, this energy is kept in a proper proportion and it's imbalance is controlled by it. A person recives only that much energy as is given by Reiki.

■■

16

Crystal Healing

Universe is affected by glorified and white light. This glorified light also affects us. White light is a collection of seven different colours which affects the seven circles (grid) of our body. Each of these seven colours is related to an important planet. This gift of nature maintains the mental and physical balance of the body, as a result, man remains hale and hearty. The central point of this light is the sun.

There is an invisible aura, one and a half inches away from our physical body. It is bright yellow in colour and acts as a link between the physical self and the cosmic power.

Aura is an important part of our life. It is invisible and represents our feelings, individuality, nature and mental capacity. Its size is that of an egg and has seven, coloured layers. Several books have been written on crystal healing all over the world, but here, I am describing it in brief.

Procedure : Light a candle or an earthen lamp in a neat and clean place. Red, pink, yellow and blue flowers (natural or artificial) are put around it. Inflame incence sticks if you are not allergic to them. Thereafter, place a quartz crystal opposite yourself, it is a symbol of all the four elements– water, fire, air and earth. Now watch the crystal in a state of peace. When your eyes start closing, close your eyes and bring the quartz crystal to the location of the third eye. Now start meditating. Do not keep the quartz crystal in that position for more than 15 minutes. It will make your third eye strong and relieve you from tension.

A quartz crystal is a good conductor and current runs through it.

Now, I will briefly describe which colour and gem is useful for which of the seven circles of the aura along with their symbol and working.

1. **Red colour** - Life giver, cures and prevents blood disorders; symbol of fire; first circle; Coral (Munga).
2. **Orange (Narangi) colour** - Symbol of energy, appetite, self control; symbol of gold; second gird; Opal.
3. **Yellow colour** - Symbol of mind and nervous system, curative for constipation and diabetes; third grid; Topaz, Ambar are useful.
4. **Green colour** - Represents sympathy, health, harmony and construction; forth grid; is useful for weak nerves, blood pressure, heart disease (yellow + blue = green i.e. when yellow and blue are mixed, it gives green); Emerald (Panna); malachite, green tyormalive are useful.
5. **Blue colour** - It gives coolness and peace; fifth grid; symbol of inspiration, will power, sacrifice and religion; Blue Lazwart, Aquamarine, Turquoise (Feroza) are useful in throat disorders.

6. **Indigo colour** - It works as a pool between decorum and wanton. It symbolises spirituality, intelligence and mystery; sixth grid; is helpful in many types of mental diseases and in the opening of the third eye.
7. **Violet colour-** In insomnia and mental problems; seventh grid; fluorite gems are useful.

YIN : For mysterious power, black tourmaline is required.

Scientific researchers, mystery investigators, doctors, etc., after performing hundreds of tests have established the remedial powers and spiritual effects of the crystal on the mind, body and emotions. For this reason, crystal healing is spreading as an alternative system of therapy.

Advantages of a Quartz Crystal :

1. As soon as a crystal comes in contact with any living thing, tree, plant, insect, animal, environment etc., the energy of that living being or thing will multiply several times.
2. Our resistance to fight diseases becomes stronger.
3. For people who believe in ghosts, sprits, evil eyes and feelings, it has an unfailing competency to protect them. It removes their bad effects and liberates them as the quartz crystal is a source of pure, spiritual energy.
4. It maintains the balance in the seven circles, thus it develops working capacity.
5. The cool nature of a quartz crystal pacifies the temper, anxiety, diseases and emotions. It removes mental and physical fatigue, providing health, peace and joy.
6. The quartz crystal protects us from the radiation and bad effects electronic machines, computers, T.V.,

tubelights etc. It absorbs all its negative effects. It also protects us form the harmful effects of atmosphere and pollution.

Method Of Using the Quartz Crystal :

To clean and endow life energy in a quartz crystal any one of the following methods canbe used.

First Method : To purify the quartz crystal, keep it drowned in sea salt for 24 hours and after that wash it with clean water.

Second Method : Keep it in sunlight for three days, the power of the quartz crystal will multiply by several folds while purifying it simultaneously.

Third Method : With pure thoughts in mind, keep the crystal in star place of worship, and jaap. The quartz crystal will become stronger.

A quartz crystal has the competence to increase wealth, food and prosperity. Experience its effects by keeping it at home and at the place of work.

For quick Relief in Pain : Seize the quartz crystal with both your hands. Keep the left hand with the quartz crystal at the place of pain and place the right hand with quartz crystal, on the rear side (opposite) of the place of pain for 15 to 20 minutes. You will get quick relief.

For treatment :

Ask the patient to hold the quartz crystal in both his hands. Make him lie down. Keep the pointed portion of the quartz crystal towards the inside of the left hand and the pointed portion of quartz crystal should be towards the out side of the right hand so that everything entering from the left hand will flow through the body and exit from the right hand, with the disease. Any other treatment if being given should be continued simultaneously, the patient will have the advantage of both the treatments.

For Immediate Relief in Anxiety, Stress, Weakness and Blood Pressure :

Keep the quartz crystal in both the hands as described above and lie down for 15-20 minutes. You will get relief at once, but while lying down imagine that the spiritual life energy is entering your body from the left hand, making your body energetic and powerful as the sickness leaves the body through the right hand.

For Quick Progress in 'Jaap' (Dhayan) :

Take two quartz crystals in both the hands, in the afore said manner. Sit down and put a wreath around your neck. This creates a quartz crystal grid around you.

To Achieve your Aim :

Watch the quartz crystal with the third eye. While concentrating on the crystal imagine that you have achieved your aim. Feel the exhilaration of success. Do it for 5 minutes and then keep the quartz crystal in your pocket, wear it in your neck or place it at your place of work. Continue this everyday till success is achieved.

For the Peace and Purity of the House :

Wherever there is a negative atmosphere or if there is a particular room, table or chair where you remain uneasy, keep a quartz crystal in that room or under the table, chair after praying (remembering God) over it. Creating four or seven quartz crystal grids is very useful. Life energy will continue to fill that room, or the area around that table or chair. This will make you feel comfortable, at ease and at peace.

In western countries, it is very much in vogue.

Miracles of Science (Dowsing)

Imagine a computer or T.V. which on the press of a button, flashes your future events, diseases, etc., then there canbe no other miracle bigger than this.

Scientists are working hard to convert this dream into reality. It is not completely impossible as 'lie detector' machines have already been invented . The whole world may treat you as 'Raja Harishchander' but, if you are guilty of lying, the machine will immediately detect it. You may pretend to lead a celebate life yet, if you have erotic dreams, then these machines can find out the time and period of such erotic dreams.

Some excellent researches are being telecast on the 'Discovery Channel' these days.

A big volume can be prepared on the achievements of science. 80% of our mind is not at all in use. The remaining 20% is also not completely used. However, our mind forecasts our past, present and future by way of our actions, photos, writings, etc. This procedure is called Dowsing. Dowsing tells us about diseases, partnership, which may be matrimonial, business or for any other purpose, who is wanting, how and how much one obeys, can be known or which of the property is movable or immovable and how much will be beneficial, can also be found out. We can get information of an enemy's army spot, and submarine, ground water, gas oil and minerals.

These machines or procedures are very much in use in Western countries.

■■

18. Insomnia (Sleeplessness)

A friend of mine suffered from insomnia. She used to take Valium 20 mg daily and is now thinking of commiting sucide even though she has no reason to do so. She has a good husband, lovely baby, a good job, a comfortable life, etc. Insomnia has disturbed her life to the extent of suicide.

Sleep is the third most important factor in life. The first two being, breathing and food. All these three are the fundamental needs of life. Disorder in any of the three, results in an imbalance. A person should give full attention to all these three fundamental needs, despite any amount of anxiety or confusion. Highs and lows are a part of life which are the result of our deeds in the previous birth or of the present one; we are helpless, we have no option but to endure them. However the present is in our hands and we should perform good deeds keeping our health and body in mind.

There are two kinds of insomnia :

1. Mental. 2. Physical.

Mental : Anxiety and fear is the cause of insomnia.

Physical : A physical disorder like cough, pain in the stomach, etc. prevents sleep.

You may see crores of people suffering from insomnia. The most common reasons are-

(1) Pondering continuously.

(2) Viewing T.V. till late at night.

(3) Excessive sleeping during daytime.

(4) Intake of liquor before sleep.

(5) Use of intoxicating medicines.

(6) Taking an unbalanced meal, at an improper time.

(7) Smoking, drinking tea or coffee before bedtime.

(8) Unknown fear.

(9) Old age.

(10) Absence or excess of sex.

Due to the excessive pollution in big cites, it is beneficial to take Vitamin C and E regularly as they help fight the bad effects of pollution in the body. We too should avoid residing in a house over which high tension electric wires pass.

Use neon lights to the minimum.

Affix a false screen on the T.V. and computer, it prevents the electronic radiations from entering our eyes.

However, the truth is that we cannot avoid electromagnetic waves. They are everywhere in a higher or lesser concentration. In other words, today we have to face the additional menace of electronic items like T.V., radios, computers, ovens, fridges, geasers, heaters, high tension wires, etc.

These radiations are absorbed by the body cells resulting in disorders and diseases like insomnia, blood

Insomnia (Sleeplessness)

cancer, etc.

We should keep a note of the undermentioned instructions for a better sleep.

1. Place should be neat and clean.
2. If not allergic to essence, the atmosphere should be fragrant.
3. Room should be airy.
4. Wear light clothes at the time of sleeping.
5. Sleep on a mattress or wooden cot. It maybe a cushion made of cotton.
6. If possible, avoid complete darkness in the room. Don't cover your mouth while sleeping.
7. Lie down straight before sleeping. Let your body loose. Take 2-3 deep breaths, keep your mind blank. Avoid thinking.
8. Remember God before going to bed.
9. People suffering from insomnia should light a candle or an earthen lamp before a picture God. Watch it peacefully for 20-30 minutes. This will help him in 3 ways :

    (a) Improve his concentration.

    (b) Enhances trust towards God.

    (c) After concentrating to 20-30 minutes, the patient experiences brainfag, his eyes became heavy and he has a sound sleep.

10. Have a light massage at night, before sleeping and then a bath. If you are unable to massage the whole body, massage your soles only. It'll induce sleep.
11. Hear soft, gentle music or read your favourite book. Avoid watching T.V. I don't mean to say that T.V. should not be viewed at all but a certain time should be fixed for watching T.V. before sleeping.

Thereafter, adopt all the above said procedures to have a sound sleep. After the fixed period of watching T.V., you should not take any sleeping pills, wine or view the T.V. again, rather you should avoid keeping the T.V. in your bedroom.

12. Don't sleep too much during the day otherwise, you will not feel sleepy in night.
13. Dinner should be a light meal.
14. If you like milk, drink luke warm milk before sleeping.
15. Do not take liquor nor advise others to take the same. But if you are addicted to liquor, take a small quantity of old wine at dinner time. New wine in a small or large quantity impairs sleep.
16. Even if you don't sleep early as a rule try to get up early in the morning. Exercise your body enough daily and regularly. Exercise will tire you and make you sleepy early, as the body demands relaxation.
17. Americans takes 150 ml to 225 ml caffeine (in tea of coffee), on an average daily, on account of which dismay, irritation, palpitations, sluggishness and insomnia like diseases begin to occur. Similarly, many people believe that alcohol stumilates our body. On the contrary it has been found to be the chief cause of anxiety and insomnia.

The quantity of caffeine in coffee, tea and soft drinks is given below :

Name.	Quantity of Caffeine in milligrams.
Coffee (7.5 oz cup)	
Drip	115-150
Brewed	80-35
Instant	40-65
Decaffeinated	3-4
Tea	
Iced	70
Soft Drink	
Coca Cola	45
Diet Coke	45
Pepsi Cola	38
Diet Pepsi	46

19 Food

The three essentials of life, as discussed earlier are breathing (oxygen) for life, food for health and sleep for relaxation. These three things are absolutely necessary to maintain our existence.

According to 'Sushruta Samahita', people should take food of every kind like sweet, pungent, salty, juicy, etc. but it should not be taken in excess. Excess of everything is bad. We should take a balanced meal and avoid imbalanced food.

You will meet certain well to do people who complain of an inability to digest food, they forget that food passes through three stages before it is ready to eat. If there is a harmony in all the three stages, only then will we be able to digest the food.

(1) **Mental state while preparing a meal :** While preparing a meal, if the cook is full of anxiety, dismay, disease, etc., then the same feelings and emotions are imbided in the meal. If food is

prepared with love and in a happy frame of mind, the food will be tasty and easily digestable.

(2) **Environment :** Atmosphere of the place where we eat food is also important. The place should be neat and clean. There should not be any bad smell, noise, etc.

(3) **Method of taking a meal :** First pay obeisance to the food and mentally utter "Oh, Annpurna, thank you for the food. I am eating now. Please continue to bless me in the future also." Don't frown at food.

If you do not like something don't speak ill of it. Eat food affectionately and do not waste. Chew the food well, otherwise it will cause flatulence.

Since times immemorial, man has worked hard and eaten fruits and roots. If we fill our stomach with pranthas, breads, cakes and heavy items without doing any hard work and exercise, an imbalance is bound to occur between the three elements and we fall ill.

Today's generation gives priority to taste. This is responsible for creating physical and mental illnesses. Parents are also responsible to some extent. They submit to the demands of their children. For example, they give tea to the child because he does not like milk. Thus the child develops the habit of drinking tea. Things harmful for children should not be placed or offered to them.

Fasting is good for health. There are multiple benefits of keeping a fast. Volumes canbe written on it. Keeping a fast once a week is good for the body. The body will feel lofty and all excretion come out of the body easily. You can adopt any of the following methods, as per your convenience :

1. Complete fast (drink only water).
2. Fast on milk (drink only milk, 2-3 times a day).

3. Fast on soup and milk (take milk in the morning and at night. Eat boiled vegetables and fruits only.).
4. Fast with one meal (take one meal during the day).

If you are unbale to keep a fast once in a week, you can fast for 7 days, twice a year during the Navratra's which is equally beneficial. Navratra's generally come in the months of April and September. These fasts not only indicate the change in season but purify the body also.

Our body consists of five elements which are (1) Akash (sky), (2) Vayu (wind), (3) Jal (water), (4) Pirthvi (earth) and (5) Agni (fire). All these elements are in equal proportions. An imbalance in either of them creates problems which is the cause of our diseases.

Country, time and circumstances also have an affect on the elements of a person. If a person from a hot country goes to cold country, he suffers from cold, cough, rheumatism, etc. Similarly, if a person from a cold country goes to a hot country, he will suffer from gastrienteritis, etc.

- You are free to eat anything that is edible, existing in this world. Eat daily but with restraint. Excess and untimely food results in disorders.
- Old wine can be taken in a little or small quantity. New wine should be avoided by daily drinkers.
- Avoid stale and dry food.
- Do not eat nik-knaks before a meal.
- Don't drink too much water while eating.
- While eating take liquids in a small quantity. But don't drink too much water or wine after a meal. Drink water 30 minutes after a meal.
- Do not over eat beyond your capacity, otherwise proper digestion will not take place.
- Chew your food well to enable prompt digestion. Do

Food

not take curd at night. If taken, mix it with cunim seed.

- Eat freshly prepared food. Avoid breads, cold drinks, tinned and packaged food.

Inappropriate Diet :

- Milk with melon, water melon, cucumber, fish, radish, wine and sour things.
- Honey with wine, hot things.
- Pork meat with hot things.
- Hot things with cold things.
- Use less of sweet syrups, butter milk and milk during the rainy season.
- Fine flour or maida should be used to the minimum.

The table given below shows the elements predominating a particular liquid:

Liquid Nature	Element	Digestive capacity		
		Vata	*Pitta*	*Kapha*
Sweet	Earth + Water	Reduces	Reduces	Increases
Alkaline	Earth + Water	Reduces	Increases	Increases
Salt	Fire + Earth	Increases	Increases	Reduces
Acidic	Fire + Air	Increases	Increases	Reduces
Sour or bitter	Sky + Air	Increases	Reduces	Reduces
Fragrant	Earth + Air	Reduces	Reduces	Reduces

Fire–Pitta–Bile

Symptom	Reason	Remedy	Disease
Offensive sweat, red face or copper pimples, constipation, good appetite, early wrinkles, impatience cracking of skin, allergy, skin diseases, premature greying of hair, hair fall.	Excess sunbathing, strong spices, condiments, food, application of hot oil (cream), use of wrong medicines or it's reaction.	Eat things which keep the belly cool such as isabgol, amla, etc. Avoid untimely and inappropriate meals. Do not take greasy and spicy food.	Jaundice, sore throat, burning in the urine, allergy, retardation, hungry in summers.

Sky–Vata–Wind–Air

Symptom	Reason	Remedy	Disease
Sleeplessness, dryness of the body, takes cold easily, peevishness, retard hunger, uneasiness, contortions of the body.	Remaining hungry for a long time, old age, lack of sleep, over indulgence in sex, eating stale and dry food.	Eating good, healthy food, reducing fat, remaining happy, a sound sleep, taking enema from time to time, take lemon-honey mixed with a little salt in a glass of water, massage with coconut oil, bath with luke warm water.	Diseases pertaining to asthma, blood dyscrasias, rheumatism, insomnia, obesity, diseases relating to digestion, mental disease.

Food

Sky–Kapha–Phelgm

Symptom	Reason	Remedy	Disease
Laziness, sleepiness, heaviness of the body, sensation of fatigue, sweet taste, sore throat, phelgm.	Salty and fried food, difficulty in digestion, reduced physical labour.	Hot food, exercise, massage with coconut oil, eating anti-kapha food materials.	Increase in kapha, lazy and sleepy, remains dull, nausea, sore throat, feels tried after least mental and physical exertion

Sphere of action of Vata, Pitta and Kapha

Wind Vata	Bile Pitta	Phelgm Kapha
Respiratory system, excretion, urine, stools, circulation of blood, functioning of the brain.	Eye, temperature of the body, appetite, thirst, glory, etc.	Body strength, semen.

Tri Doshas	Vata	Pitta	Kapha
Rainy season	More	Less	Less
Summer & Autumn	−	+	−
Winter	−	−	+
Childhood	−	−	+
Adolescence	+	−	−
Old age	+	−	−
Jungle	+	−	−
Sandy area (desert)	+	+	−
Gulf, bay (Khari)	−	+	+
Hilly area	+	−	+
Plain area	+	+	+
6 A.M. to 10 A.M.	−	−	+
10 A.M. to 14 P.M.	−	+	−
14 P.M. to 18 P.M.	+	−	−
18 P.M. to 22 A.M.	−	−	+
22 P.M. to 2 A.M.	−	+	−
2 A.M. to 6 A.M.	+	−	−
		+ More	− Less.

The following chart gives you information regarding the sugar content in various eatables. Patients should, consume food items with more carbohydrates and sugar

Sugar	Vegetables	Cereals
Glucose-100	Beets-64	Bran cereal-59
Maltas-105	Carrot-31	Bread, white-69
Honey-75	Cooked carrot-36	Whole grain-72
Sucrose-60	Fried potato-98	Maize-59
Fructose-20	Potato (fresh boiled) −70	Corn flakes-80

Food

Fruits	Other Eatables	Oatmeals
Apple	Ice cream-36	Pistachio-45
Banana	Milk-34	Rice-70
Orange	Nuts-13	Rice, puffed-95
Raisin	Beans-31	Grains-67
Orange juice	Lentils-29	
	Peas-39.	

Food Allergy

There are two main reasons for food allergies. One is improper digestion and the other is feeling tired and anxious. Starch and edible, permitted colours do not suit some people. Allergy can occur on account of some proteins also. Pollution also causes food allergy. Air, water and environment pollution has a great effect. Pollution is also caused by T.Vs, computers, electric lights and electronic items. Giving solid food to tinytots before age also causes an allergy.

We can determine our food or respiratory allergies by three ways:

1. Presence of black circles below the eyes.
2. Inflammation below the eyes.
3. Inflammation of glands (adenitis).

How to perform a test for food allergy.

It can be done by two ways:

(1) Food challenge.
(2) By testing in a laboratory.

Food challenge test can be done at home without any cost, but a lot of care has to be taken and it should be done according to the rules. Laboratory tests, are costly but results are immediate.

Food Challenge Test :

1. First of all, we should see which food causes heaviness, distaste or creates flatulence, whether it is vegetarian or non-vegetarian, solid or liquid. Prepare a list of such food articles and avoid eating them for a month. After one month, start eating them again. If they again disagree with you, it means they are causing an allergy. Consult a doctor for permanent treatment.

2. Use mineral or boiled water.

3. Old people should not try the food challenge test, the allergy after a month may become severe causing detrimental problems. They should directly seek help of a laboratory or doctor.

Main thing to be noted is that you have to quit all those food articles which cause an allergy or tend to cause an allergy. If you quit rice then you also have to quit it's allied products. One kind of food and it's allies (whether vegetarian or non-vegetarian) are counted under one food family.

Symptoms and diseases caused by food allergy are :

Intestinal : Diarrhea, flatus, ulcer, etc.

Genito–urinary : Bed wetting, bladder and kidney infection, etc.

Immunity : Chronic infections, ear infections.

Mental / Emotional : Anxiety, depression, insomnia, irritation, loss of concentration, etc.

Respiratory : Asthma, chronic bronchitis, wheezing, etc.

Skin : Ring worm, itching, eczema.

Others : Backache, joint pains, ear, nose, throat infection, headache, tiredness, epilepsy, etc.

Food

Description of food families veg and non veg.

Legumes	Mustard	Parsley	Potato
Beans	Brocolli	Anis	Chili
Cocabeans	Brussel	Caraway	Eggplant
Lentils	Cabbage	Carrot	Pepper
Peanuts	Mustard	celary	Potato
Soyabeans	Radish	Corriander	Tobacco
Peas	Turnip	Cagamin	Tomato
--	Sprout	--	--

Gross	Lily	Lorel	Semflower
Barley	Asparagus	Avocado	Antichoke
Corn	Cheese	Camphor	Lotus
Oat	Garlic	Chinamin	Semflower
Rice	Lincus	--	--
Wheat	Onion	--	--

Fruits:

Grapes	Pineapple	Papaya	Apple
Grape	Pineapple	Papaya	Pear
Raisin	--	--	Apple

Gourds	Plums	Citrus	Cashew
Cantaloupe	Almond	Grape fruit	Cashew
Cucumber	Apricot	Lemon	Mango
--	Cherry	Lime	Pistachio
Melons	Peach	--	--
Pumpkin	--	Orange	--
Squash	Plum	--	--

Nuts	Beach	Banana	Palm
Brazil Nut	Beechnut	Arrowroot	Coconut
Wall Nut	Chestnut	Banana	Date
Peekins	Chinqapin	Plaintain	Date Sugar.

Rose	Blueberry	
Blackberry	Blueberry.	
Loganberry	Cranberry	
Raspberry	Huckleberry.	
Rose Hips	--	
Strawberry	--	

Milk	Meat/Egg
Cow	Goat
Goat	Pig
Camel	Rabbit
Sheep	Sheep
--	Chicken
--	Duck
--	Hen
--	Turkey

Fish	Crustaceans	Molluscs
Catfish	Crab	--
Tuna	Crayfish	Oyesters
Snapper	Lobster	Mussels
Sardine	Prawn	Scallops
Salmon	--	--
Cad	--	--
Flounder	--	--
Helibeat	--	--

For the last 20-25 years, incidence of food allergies has been increasing in a dramatic manner. Sixty percent people are affected by food allergies in America only.

The following chart shows the symptoms and diseases due to food allergy.

Nutritional composition (Quantity in gram):

List	Protein	Fat	Carbohy-derates	Fibre	Colories
Vegetable	3	0	11	1-3	50
Fruits	0	0	20	1-3	80
Breads, etc.	2	0	15	1-4	70
Legumes	7	0.5	15	6-7	90
Fats	0	5	0	0	45
Milk	8	0	12	–	80
Meat, etc.	7	3	0	0	55

Height and Weight Table:

The following chart shows us how much weight a man/woman should have, in accordance to their height. Weight is shown in lbs (pounds):

Men		Women	
Height	Weight	Height	Weight
5' – 2"	131 – 141	4' – 10"	109 – 121
5' – 3"	133 – 143	4' – 11"	111 – 123
5' – 4"	135 – 145	5' – 00"	113 – 126
5' – 5"	137 – 148	5' – 1"	115 – 119
5' – 6"	139 – 151	5' – 2"	118 – 132
		5 – 3"	121 – 135

Men		Women	
Height	Weight	Height	Weight
5' – 7"	142 – 154	5' – 4"	124 – 138
5' – 8"	145 – 157	5' – 5"	127 – 141
5' – 9"	148 – 160	5' – 6"	130 – 144
5' – 10"	151 – 163	5' – 7"	133 – 147
5' – 11"	154 – 166	5' – 8"	136 – 150
6' – 00"	157 – 170	5' – 9"	139 – 153
6' – 1"	160 – 174	5' – 10"	142 – 156
6' – 2"	164 – 178	5' – 11"	142 – 159
6' – 3"	167 – 182	6' – 00"	148 – 162
6' – 4"	171 – 187	--	--

Chart showing quantity of the three Tri Doshas in vegetables, cereals, etc.

Name	Vata Wind	Pitta Bile	Kapha Phelgm
Kidney bean	=	=	=
Horse bean	−	+	+
Lentil seed	+	−	−
Green peanuts	+	−	−
Potato	+	+	+
Gram	=	=	=
Soyabean	−	+	+
Spinach	+	−	−
Cabbage	+	−	−
Cauliflower	+	+	−
Brinjal	+	+	+
Lady's finger	−	−	+
Beans	+	+	+
Tomato	+	−	−
Radish	=	=	=
Radish leaves	+	+	
Carrot	=	=	=
Turnip	=	=	=
Bittergourd	=	=	=
Orange	−	+	−
Lemon	−	+	−
Apple	−	−	+
Sour apple	−	+	+
Banana	−	−	+
Banana, ripe	+	−	+
Grapes	=	=	=
Sour grapes	−	+	−
Mango	=	=	=
Peach	−	+	−
Litchi	−	+	+
Pear	−	−	+

Food

Name	Vata Wind	Pitta Bile	Kapha Phelgm
Pomegranate	=	=	=
Date fruit	−	+	+
Guava	+	−	+
Musk melon	−	+	+
Water melon	−	+	+
Pineapple	−	+	+
Fig	−	+	−
Almond	−	+	+
Pistachio	−	+	+
Cherongi	−	+	+
Cashewnut	−	+	+
Walnut	−	+	+
Milk	=	=	=
Curd	−	+	+
Cheese	−	±	±
Ghee	−	−	+
Butter	−	−	+
Egg	−	+	+
Fish	+	−	+
Mutton	−	−	+
Goat	−	−	−
Pig	−	+	+
Horse	−	+	+
Deer	=	=	=
Cock	−	+	+
Wild cock	−	−	+
Tea / coffee	+	±	+
Honey	−	+	−
Sugar	−	+	+
Edible oil	−	+	−
Anisseed	−	−	+
Cardamon (green)	=	=	=
Cardomon (brown)	−	+	−
Cinnamon	−	+	−

Name	Vata Wind	Pitta Bile	Kapha Phelgm
Mulhati	=	=	=
Cumin seeds	−	+	−
Carraway	−	+	−
Corriander	=	=	=
Fenugreek	−	+	+
Soya	−	+	−
Kalonji	−	+	−
Clove	−	+	−
Basil	−	+	−
Turmeric	=	=	=
Neem	+	−	−
Peeple	+	−	−
Ginger	−	+	−
Garlic	−	+	−
Asafoetida	−	+	−
Nutmeg	−	+	−
Mustard seed	−	+	−
Black pepper	−	+	−

20

Flower Therapy

If you are disappointed by other systems of medicines and fed up of your illness, then try Flower Therapy, which will find your hidden disease and emotion, and will make you perfectly normal.

My mother was suffering from sciatica. My first experiment with Flower therapy was on my family. She had taken a lot of medicines and injections, but all failed. Allopathy, gave here immediate but temporary relief. Ayurvedic therapy claimed to cure her but over a long period of time, she consulted 2-3 vaids but was not benefited by any. Homoeopathy gave relief but she could not take the preventive measures advocated by the homoeopath. She had pain throughout the night. Finally she tried Flower therapy, which cured 80% of her ailment. She is still taking the same therapy.

There are certain things, habits and nature, which doctors cannot treat, for example, insomnia, jealousy, inferiority complex, etc. They cannot make a man kind hearted or remove his fear, stress, weakness in studies, etc.

As the root cause of disease lies in the mind, Dr. Bach prescribes on the basis of mental and emotional symptoms, and habits of the patient.

To achieve this, Dr. Bach took the help of nature. He observed that flowers, although sensitive, bear all attacks or blows of nature, and yet they blossom. Every flower has it's own effect, influence and power. He selected 38 flowers having different influences and made an essence from them. We can take 2-3 essences and mix them together if the case demands.

For example, use Mimulus in treating fear, give Pine to an irritated person. Scloranthus should be given to a person with the habit of forgetting. To treat intolerance and jealousy, Beech is prescribed. Take Horn bean for power, etc.

Dr. Bach left for the heavenly abode in 1936 but his alternate therapy has created a major impact on the world. This therapy is popular in America, Germany, Australia, Switzerland and England.

Flower therapy has treatment for all the above mentioned disorders and this therapy has no adverse effect of any kind, nor does it clash with any other therapy. Although, it's effect is reduced if allopathic medicines are taken simultaneously.

Dr. Bach introduced the Flower therapy and thus it is also known as Bach's Flower Therapy.

Dr. Bach was posted at the University College Hospital, London as a bacteriologist. He was also a medical officer there for sometime. After resigning from the post, he started a private practice. He was not satisfied with the allopathic mode of treatment. He felt that allopathy did not eradicate the disease from the root. According to him the root cause of all diseases lies in our mind. If we are irritated, tense or afraid, hindrances are created in our nervous system and they block the smooth flow of impulses which can create diseases and also enhance them. If these obstructions are removed, diseases vanish.

21

Summary

Three principles :

1. Keep three things in mind while testing a person.

   (1) His behaviour.

   (2) His nature.

   (3) His family.

   If he is found unadulterated in all three things, then we need no guarantee. Otherwise even God's guarantee will not do any good.

2. Observe three rules for a life long partnership:

   (1) Punctuality.

   (2) Keeping the accounts properly.

   (3) Do not take partnership money for your own or personal use.

3. To make a person yours:

   (1) Do not expect anything from him.

   (2) Do not give false promises or assurance

(3) Observe good mannerisms.

Three principles for health :

(1) Exercise Pranayam and massage once in a week.
(2) Do not eat unnutritions meals. Eat with respect and masticate each morsel thoroughly before swallowing it.
(3) Drink maximum water.

Intrinsic three principles :

(1) Never be disappointed. Instead of worrying, meditate.
(2) Always be optimistic.
(3) Believe in God.

Last three principles :

(1) Do not meddle with the affairs of others.
(2) Do not peep into others life.
(3) Do not compete.

Miracles by alternate therapy :

Two third of the diseases (except contageous disease) occur on account of stress and tension like ulcers, diabetes, cancer, rheumatism, insomnia, hypertension, heart disease, disorders of the nervous system, etc. We can cure tension, loss of memory, power, etc. by alternate therapy. Now a days this alternative therapy is gaining popularity all over the world.

Reiki :

It is a Japanese therapy which means universal life giving energy. If energy functions properly in our body, we will remain healthy. If any block is created then we will be afflicted with mental and physical disorders. If we loose all the energy from our body, we will become cold i.e. dead.

Reiki can be given to any animal, tree or person. It makes a person optimistic.

Magnified Healing :

It is over and above Reiki but it's procedure is like that of Reiki.

Flower Therapy :

Tension and nature both are responsible for diseases. If we treat the patient by analysing his nature, cure is achieved. It is capable in treating all diseases. It was invented in U.K. Essence of flowers is used to treat patients. It has no adverse effects. All mental and physical diseases are cured permanently by it.

Crystal and Pyramid Healing :

It is an European therapy. Quartz crystal is the best medium to absorb energy. 'Pyra' means energy and 'Mid' means centre. Pyramid also draws energy from the top and makes animate and inanimate life longer.

Indian Aurvedic Massage :

If you don't have time for yoga and are a case of insomnia, try taking a massage daily. See the effects yourself.

Scientific Numbering :

If we can change the order of time, we can also change the horoscope of a person. But dates of birth are permanent in case you are sure of your birth date, then you can find out :

(1) The nature of your husband to be.

Summary

(2) Assessment of yours and your firm's name.
(3) Health, position, etc
(4) Desires, colours, etc.

Dowsing :

It is also an European therapy. Through Dowsing we can know where the disorder in the body is, answers to question arising in our mind regarding partnership, matrimony, business, etc. canbe answered by it. It can be performed on the person himself in a better way or by examining his writing, photograph, etc.